T0210246

Diagnostic Excellence in the ICU: Thinking Critically and Masterfully

Editors

PAUL A. BERGL
RAHUL S. NANCHAL

CRITICAL CARE CLINICS

www.criticalcare.theclinics.com

Consulting Editor
GREGORY S. MARTIN

January 2022 • Volume 38 • Number 1

ELSEVIER

1600 John F. Kennedy Boulevard • Suite 1800 • Philadelphia, Pennsylvania, 19103-2899

http://www.theclinics.com

CRITICAL CARE CLINICS Volume 38, Number 1
January 2022 ISSN 0749-0704, ISBN-13: 978-0-323-81339-6

Editor: Joanna Collett
Developmental Editor: Hannah Almira Lopez

Critical Care Clinics (ISSN: 0749-0704) is published quarterly by Elsevier Inc., 360 Park Avenue South, New York, NY 10010-1710. Months of issue are January, April, July, and October. Business and Editorial Offices: 1600 John F. Kennedy Blvd., Suite 1800, Philadelphia, PA 19103-2899. Customer Service Office: 6277 Sea Harbor Drive, Orlando, FL 32887-4800. Periodicals postage paid at New York, NY and additional mailing offices. Subscription prices are $266.00 per year for US individuals, $921.00 per year for US institutions, $100.00 per year for US students and residents, $296.00 per year for Canadian individuals, $953.00 per year for Canadian institutions, $338.00 per year for international individuals, $953.00 per year for international institutions, $100.00 per year for Canadian students/residents, and $150.00 per year for foreign students/residents. To receive student/resident rate, orders must be accompanied by name of affiliated institution, date of term, and the signature of program/residency coordinator on institution letterhead. Orders will be billed at individual rate until proof of status is received. Foreign air speed delivery is included in all *Clinics* subscription prices. All prices are subject to change without notice. POSTMASTER: Send address changes to *Critical Care Clinics*, Elsevier Periodicals Customer Service, 11830 Westline Industrial Drive, St. Louis, MO 63146. **Customer Service: 1-800-654-2452 (US). From outside of the US, call 1-314-447-8871. Fax: 1-314-447-8029. E-mail: journalscustomerservice-usa@elsevier.com (for print support) or journalsonlinesupport-usa@elsevier.com (for online support).**

Reprints. For copies of 100 or more of articles in this publication, please contact the Commercial Reprints Department, Elsevier Inc., 360 Park Avenue South, New York, NY 10010-1710. Tel.: 212-633-3874; Fax: 212-633-3820; E-mail: reprints@elsevier.com.

Critical Care Clinics is also published in Spanish by Editorial Inter-Medica, Junin 917, 1er A, 1113, Buenos Aires, Argentina.

Critical Care Clinics is covered in *MEDLINE/PubMed (Index Medicus), EMBASE/Excerpta Medica, Current Concepts/Clinical Medicine, ISI/BIOMED, and Chemical Abstracts.*

Contributors

CONSULTING EDITOR

GREGORY S. MARTIN, MD, MSC
Professor, Division of Pulmonary, Allergy, Critical Care and Sleep Medicine, Research Director, Emory Critical Care Center, Director, Emory/Georgia Tech Predictive Health Institute, Co-Director, Atlanta Center for Microsystems Engineered Point-of-Care Technologies (ACME POCT), President, Society of Critical Care Medicine, Atlanta, Georgia

EDITORS

PAUL A. BERGL, MD
Intensivist, Department of Critical Care, Gundersen Lutheran Medical Center, La Crosse, Wisconsin; Clinical Adjunct Assistant Professor, Department of Medicine, University of Wisconsin School of Medicine and Public Health, Madison, Wisconsin

RAHUL S. NANCHAL, MD
Professor of Medicine, Division of Pulmonary and Critical Care Medicine, Hub for Collaborative Medicine, Practicing Intensivist, Department of Medicine, Medical College of Wisconsin, Milwaukee, Wisconsin

AUTHORS

GOPI J. ASTIK, MD, MS
Assistant Professor of Medicine, Division of Hospital Medicine, Northwestern University Feinberg School of Medicine, Chicago, Illinois

MARK BARASH, DO
Assistant Professor of Medicine, Division of Pulmonary and Critical Care Medicine, Hub for Collaborative Medicine, Medical College of Wisconsin, Milwaukee, Wisconsin

PAUL A. BERGL, MD
Intensivist, Department of Critical Care, Gundersen Lutheran Medical Center, La Crosse, Wisconsin; Clinical Adjunct Assistant Professor, Department of Medicine, University of Wisconsin School of Medicine and Public Health, Madison, Wisconsin

MEGAN CHRISTENSON, MD, MPH
Department of Medicine, Division of Pulmonary and Critical Care Medicine, Medical College of Wisconsin, Milwaukee, Wisconsin

CHRISTINA L. CIFRA, MD, MS
Clinical Associate Professor, Division of Critical Care, Department of Pediatrics, University of Iowa Carver College of Medicine, Iowa City, Iowa

JASON W. CUSTER, MD
Associate Professor, Division of Critical Care, Department of Pediatrics, University of Maryland, Baltimore, Maryland; Medical Director of Patient Safety, University of Maryland Medical Center, Baltimore, Maryland

ROBERT EL-KAREH, MD, MPH, MS
Associate Professor of Medicine, University of California, San Diego, La Jolla, California

JAMES C. FACKLER, MD
Associate Professor, Division of Pediatric Anesthesia and Critical Care, Department of Anesthesiology and Critical Care Medicine, Johns Hopkins School of Medicine, Baltimore, Maryland; Johns Hopkins Charlotte R. Bloomberg Children's Center, Baltimore, Maryland

YASAMAN FATEMI, MD
Division of Infectious Diseases, Children's Hospital of Philadelphia, Philadelphia, Pennsylvania

KANEKAL SURESH GAUTHAM, MD, DM, MS, FAAP
Pediatrician-in-Chief, Nemours Children's Hospital, Orlando, Florida

EMILY HARRIS, MD
Internal Medicine Resident, University of California San Francisco, San Francisco, California

PRASHANT MAHAJAN, MD, MPH, MBA
Professor, Departments of Emergency Medicine and Pediatrics, University of Michigan, Ann Arbor, Michigan

COURTNEY W. MANGUS, MD
Instructor, Departments of Emergency Medicine and Pediatrics, University of Michigan, Ann Arbor, Michigan

RAHUL S. NANCHAL, MD, MS
Professor of Medicine, Division of Pulmonary and Critical Care Medicine, Hub for Collaborative Medicine, Practicing Intensivist, Department of Medicine, Medical College of Wisconsin, Milwaukee, Wisconsin

ANDREW P.J. OLSON, MD
Associate Professor of Medicine, Department of Medicine and Pediatrics, University of Minnesota Medical School, Minneapolis, Minnesota

JAYSHIL J. PATEL, MD
Department of Medicine, Division of Pulmonary and Critical Care Medicine, Medical College of Wisconsin, Milwaukee, Wisconsin

JEREMY B. RICHARDS, MD, MA
Assistant Professor of Medicine, Division of Pulmonary, Critical Care, and Sleep Medicine, Beth Israel Deaconess Medical Center, Boston, Massachusetts

LEKSHMI SANTHOSH, MD, MAEd
Assistant Professor of Pulmonary and Critical Care Medicine, University of California San Francisco, San Francisco, California

RICHARD M. SCHWARTZSTEIN, MD
Professor of Medicine, Division of Pulmonary, Critical Care, and Sleep Medicine, Beth Israel Deaconess Medical Center, Boston, Massachusetts

GRANT SHAFER, MD, MA, FAAP
Neonatologist, Division of Neonatology, Children's Hospital of Orange County, Orange, California

ANUJ SHUKLA, MD
Department of Medicine, Division of Pulmonary and Critical Care Medicine, Medical College of Wisconsin, Milwaukee, Wisconsin

DEAN F. SITTIG, PhD
Professor, School of Biomedical Informatics, The University of Texas Health Science Center at Houston, UT-Memorial Hermann Center for Healthcare Quality & Safety, Houston, Texas

YAN ZHOU, MD
Intensivist, Department of Critical Care Medicine, Geisinger Medical Center, Danville, Pennsylvania; Clinical Assistant Professor, Geisinger Commonwealth School of Medicine, Scranton, Pennsylvania

Contents

cognitive biases, which can lead to diagnostic errors. A variety of strategies have been proposed to mitigate biases; however, current understanding of such interventions to optimize diagnostic safety is still incomplete.

Clinical reasoning is prone to errors in judgment. Error is comprised of 2 components—bias and noise; each has an equally important role in the promulgation of error. Biases or systematic errors in reasoning are the product of misconceptions of probability and statistics. Biases arise because clinicians frequently rely on mental shortcuts or heuristics to make judgments. The most frequently used heuristics are representativeness, availability, and anchoring/adjustment which lead to the common biases of base rate neglect, misconceptions of regression, insensitivities to sample size, and fallacies of conjunctive, and disjunctive events. Bayesian reasoning is the framework within which posterior probabilities of events is identified. Familiarity with these mathematical concepts will likely enhance clinical reasoning. Noise is defined as inter or intraobserver variability in judgment that should be identical. Guidelines in medicine are a technique to reduce noise.

Diagnostic stewardship encompasses the entire diagnosis-to-treatment paradigm in the intensive care unit (ICU). Initially born of the antimicrobial stewardship movement, contemporary diagnostic stewardship aims to promote timely and appropriate diagnostic testing that directly links to management decisions. In the stewardship framework, excessive diagnostic testing in low probability cases is discouraged due to its tendency to generate false-positive results, which have their own downstream consequences. Though the evidence basis for diagnostic stewardship initiatives in the ICU is nascent and largely limited to retrospective analyses, available literature generally suggests that these initiatives are safe, feasible, and associated with similar patient outcomes. As diagnostic testing of critically ill patients becomes increasingly sophisticated in the ensuing decade, a stewardship mindset will aid bedside clinicians in interpreting and incorporating new diagnostic strategies in the ICU.

Diagnostic errors are considered a blind spot of health care delivery and occur in up to 15% of patient cases. Cognitive failures are a leading cause of diagnostic error and often occur as a result of overreliance on system 1 thinking. This narrative review describes why diagnostic errors occur by shedding additional light on systems 1 and 2 forms of thinking, reviews literature on debiasing strategies in medicine, and provides a framework for teaching critical thinking in the intensive care unit as a strategy to promote learner development and minimize cognitive failures.

Identification of diagnostic errors is difficult but is not alone sufficient for performance improvement. Instead, cases must be reflected on to identify ways to improve decision-making in the future. There are many tools and modalities to retrospectively reflect on action to study medical decisions and outcomes and improve future performance. Reflection in action—in which diagnostic decisions are considered in real-time—may also improve medical decision-making especially through strategies such as structured reflection. Ongoing regular feedback can normalize the discussion about improving decision-making, enable reflective practice, and improve decision making.

Effective and efficient critical thinking skills are necessary to engage in accurate clinical reasoning and to make appropriate clinical decisions. Teaching and promoting critical thinking skills in the intensive care unit is challenging because of the volume of data and the constant distractions of competing obligations. Understanding and acknowledging cognitive biases and their impact on clinical reasoning are necessary to promote and support critical thinking in the ICU. Active educational strategies such as concept or mechanism mapping can help to diagnose disorganized thinking and reinforce key connections and important clinical and pathophysiologic concepts, which are critical for inductive reasoning.

Patient care in intensive care environments is complex, time-sensitive, and data-rich, factors that make these settings particularly well-suited to clinical decision support (CDS). A wide range of CDS interventions have been used in intensive care unit environments. The field needs well-designed studies to identify the most effective CDS approaches. Evolving artificial intelligence and machine learning models may reduce information-overload and enable teams to take better advantage of the large volume of patient data available to them. It is vital to effectively integrate new CDS into clinical workflows and to align closely with the cognitive processes of frontline clinicians.

Diagnosing critically ill patients in the intensive care unit is difficult. As a result, diagnostic errors in the intensive care unit are common and have been shown to cause harm. Research to improve diagnosis in critical care medicine has accelerated in past years. However, much work remains to fully elucidate the diagnostic process in critical care. To achieve diagnostic excellence, interdisciplinary research is needed, adopting a balanced strategy of continued biomedical discovery while addressing the complex care delivery systems underpinning the diagnosis of critical illness.

CRITICAL CARE CLINICS

SERIES OF RELATED INTEREST

Hematology/Oncology Clinics
https://www.hemonc.theclinics.com/

THE CLINICS ARE AVAILABLE ONLINE!
Access your subscription at:
www.theclinics.com

Preface

The Quest for Diagnostic Excellence in Critical Care

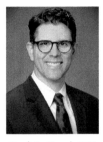 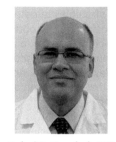

Paul A. Bergl, MD   Rahul S. Nanchal, MD

Editors

The modern intensive care unit (ICU) abounds with complexity. We support multiple failing organ systems, often among patients with a bewildering array of comorbidities and complications. We deal with the challenging tripartite intersection of what is possible, what patients and families desire, and what is reasonable. To stabilize deranged physiology, we apply an armamentarium of sophisticated technologies that in turn generate patient data ad infinitum: vital signs, laboratory test results, diagnostic images, ventilator parameters, measures of cardiac output, fluid balances, and much more.

This immense body of patient data notwithstanding, we as intensivists face significant challenges in arriving at accurate diagnoses for our critically ill patients. Our patients often cannot provide a cogent history of their illness, and we must rely on imperfect information provided second or third hand. Furthermore, by the time a patient arrives in the ICU, they usually have been subjected to a number of interventions that affect their physiology, change the natural history of their illness, and muddy our own judgment. We practice at a brisk pace, and the cognitively taxing nature of our work is compounded by the high stakes of stabilizing patients on the brink of death and the charged emotions that emanate from our patients, families, staff, and colleagues.

Unsurprisingly, the labyrinthian and stressful ICU environment is rife with errors in judgment and diagnosis. Reasonable estimates suggest that at least 5% of deaths in the ICU result from fatal misdiagnoses. Nonfatal diagnostic errors, which occur in an additional 5% to 10% of ICU patients, also confer significant morbidity, generate immense financial costs, and have heavy emotional tolls.

This issue of the *Critical Care Clinics* explores diagnostic excellence in the ICU from various perspectives. Because discussing the topic requires a shared dialect and foundational knowledge, we first review definitions of diagnostic errors, methods for

Crit Care Clin 38 (2022) xi–xii
https://doi.org/10.1016/j.ccc.2021.09.004
0749-0704/22/© 2021 Published by Elsevier Inc.

criticalcare.theclinics.com

identifying them, and the epidemiology of diagnostic error in critical care. We then delve into the science of human cognition and provide a contemporary understanding of how intensivists arrive at a diagnosis and the pitfalls that lead to reasoning errors.

In the latter half of this issue, we propose potential solutions to mitigate errors and to promote diagnostic excellence in the ICU. We introduce the concept of diagnostic stewardship and examine how systems can be designed to improve the appropriateness, and accordingly, the utility and accuracy, of diagnostic testing. We then return to human cognition and discuss practical strategies and educational interventions to improve diagnostic reasoning. Building upon strategies targeted at improving individual clinician's diagnostic performance, we consider how to optimize teamwork and ultimately how to reengineer our health care delivery systems to improve diagnosis. We discuss how structured reflection, feedback, and routine diagnostic auditing could operate at both the individual and the systems level of care to reduce cognitive failures. Finally, we conclude with a research agenda that hones in on aspects of our care delivery systems that affect the diagnostic process.

Diagnostic errors remain unacceptably common in the ICU. We hope that this issue of *Critical Care Clinics* will galvanize the critical care community to develop pragmatic solutions to this neglected area of patient safety. Our patients deserve the safest, most-effective care possible; diagnostic excellence is the backbone of such care.

Paul A. Bergl, MD
Gundersen Lutheran Medical Center
1900 South Avenue, Mail Stop LM3-001
La Crosse, WI 54601, USA

Rahul S. Nanchal, MD
Medical College of Wisconsin
Division of Pulmonary, Critical Care, and Sleep Medicine
8th Floor, Hub for Collaborative Medicine
8701 West Watertown Plank Road
Milwaukee, WI 53226, USA

E-mail addresses:
pabergl@gundersenhealth.org (P.A. Bergl)
rnanchal@mcw.edu (R.S. Nanchal)

Diagnostic Error: Why Now?

Grant Shafer, MD, MA[a],*, Kanekal Suresh Gautham, MD, DM, MS[b]

KEYWORDS

- Diagnosis • Diagnostic error • Patient safety • Quality • Intensive care unit
- Critical care • National Academy of Medicine

KEY POINTS

- Diagnostic error remains challenging to define and quantify in medicine.
- Despite concerted efforts over the years, a singular, encompassing definition of diagnostic error has yet to be identified.
- A variety of methodologies have been used to measure diagnostic error, but there is currently no widely accepted approach to quantification.
- The 2015 report by the National Academy of Medicine remains a sentinel publication for the diagnostic error movement and contains key explanations and recommendations.

INTRODUCTION

The groundbreaking 1999 report, *To Err Is Human: Building a Safer Health System*, by the Institute of Medicine (now the National Academy of Medicine, or NAM) galvanized the modern patient safety movement, which led to widespread, concerted efforts to measure, understand, and address errors in medicine.[1–3] Despite the significant advances made by the patient safety movement, however, the focus has centered primarily on errors in treatment, such as medication administration, hospital-acquired infections, and wrong-site surgery, and as a result, diagnostic errors remain relatively understudied and unmeasured.[4–9] The reasons for this lag are multifactorial: lack of effective instruments to measure diagnostic errors, complex and multifaceted causes, disagreement as to what constitutes a diagnostic error, and less obvious solutions to this problem in comparison to other types of error.[2,5,6,8]

Fortunately, there has been an increasing awareness of the importance of diagnostic errors, and of the need to make progress in this area.[5] Although limitations in the measurement of diagnostic error have led to difficulty in defining the full scope of the problem, the available data highlight its pervasive nature. Estimates indicate diagnostic errors occur in 5% of adult outpatient encounters annually and account

[a] Division of Neonatology, Children's Hospital of Orange County, 1201 West La Veta Avenue, Orange, CA 92868, USA; [b] Nemours Children's Hospital, 6535 Nemours Parkway, Orlando, FL 32827, USA
* Corresponding author.
E-mail address: grant.shafer@choc.org
Twitter: @shafergt (G.S.)

Crit Care Clin 38 (2022) 1–10
https://doi.org/10.1016/j.ccc.2021.08.001
0749-0704/22/© 2021 Elsevier Inc. All rights reserved.

for 6% to 17% of all hospital adverse events, and the NAM predicts that most people will experience at least 1 diagnostic error in their lifetime.[2,7] The significance of this trend is amplified in the intensive care unit (ICU), where as many as 40,500 adult patients in the United States may die annually from a diagnostic error.[10]

As the significance of diagnostic errors and the continued lag in their study and prevention became apparent, the NAM released a follow-up report in 2015, *Improving Diagnosis in Healthcare,* to address the need for more emphasis on errors in diagnosis.[2] This comprehensive undertaking summarized the problem of diagnostic errors, acknowledged that diagnostic errors continue to harm an unacceptable number of patients, and emphasized that improving the diagnostic process remains a moral, professional, and public health imperative.[2] This call to action has been corroborated by other organizations who have spoken out on the need to decrease the harm caused by diagnostic errors. The World Health Organization recently listed diagnostic errors as 1 of the 5 "high-priority" causes of patient safety incidents.[11] In the 2018, 2019, and 2020 editions of their annual executive brief, "Top 10 Patient Safety Concerns," the Emergency Care Research Institute (ECRI) listed diagnostic errors as the number one priority for the year.[12–14] The ECRI also posits that some negative outcomes that were previously attributed to the natural course of disease may in fact have been due to diagnostic errors.[15]

The slow progress in the understanding of the incidence and nature of diagnostic errors as well as the lack of high-quality evidence on how to prevent these errors is especially critical in the ICU. Patients in critical care settings are particularly vulnerable to preventable harm from diagnostic errors, which tend be more lethal with increased acuity of patient illness.[16–20] Increasing the understanding of the incidence and cause of diagnostic error in critical care could potentially decrease preventable harm in the ICU.[21]

In this article, the authors explore some of the controversies in defining diagnostic error and review current methods of detection and measurement. They also summarize key points and recommendations from the seminal NAM report, *Improving Diagnosis in Healthcare.*

DEFINITION

A primary barrier to the study of errors in diagnosis has been the difficulty in conceptualizing an encompassing, functional definition for diagnostic error. Diagnosis is a complex process that unfolds over time within the setting of the health care system; as a result, it is often difficult to quantify.[2] The diagnostic process involves the complex interaction among a patient experiencing a health problem, the health care system, health care professionals who gather and process diagnostic information to determine a likely diagnosis, and subsequent communication of this diagnostic reasoning back to the patient. This complex interaction is summarized by the NAM in **Fig. 1**.

Unfortunately, the diagnostic process in the ICU, similar to other dynamic, rapidly paced settings, is often not so linear. Critically ill patients may present in active deterioration, which forces the intensivist to prioritize stabilization over a formal diagnostic evaluation. Furthermore, the rapidly changing physiology of a deteriorating patient may force the clinician to simultaneously attempt to determine the cause of illness while treating emergent clinical conditions. This may include a large amount of data being obtained at the same time as life-saving stabilization measures are being performed. In situations whereby deterioration outpaces resuscitative efforts, the intensivist may be required to pause diagnostic endeavors entirely in order to focus on

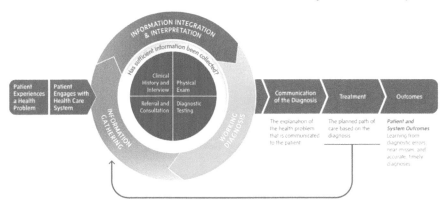

Fig. 1. The diagnostic process. (National Academies of Sciences, Engineering, and Medicine. 2015. Improving Diagnosis in Health Care. Washington, DC: The National Academies Press. https://doi.org/10.17226/21794. Reproduced with permission from the National Academy of Sciences, Courtesy of the National Academies Press, Washington, D.C.)

life-saving interventions. The complex and nonlinear diagnostic process in the ICU is summarized by Bergl and colleagues in **Fig. 2**.[16]

Given the intricacies of this process, there are sometimes breakdowns leading to errors in diagnosis. The NAM defines a medical error as "failure of a planned action to be completed as intended (error of execution) and the use of a wrong plan to achieve an aim (error of planning)" or "failure of a planned action that should have been completed (omission)."[22] Errors can lead to adverse events or "events that result in unintended harm to the patient by an act of commission or omission rather than by the underlying disease or condition of the patient."[22]

A major difficulty in conceptualizing an operational definition of diagnostic error is the disagreement in what constitutes a diagnostic error. This controversy stems in part from the fact that the term "diagnosis" can refer to both a process and the end outcome of the process.[23] Some consider a diagnostic error and misdiagnosis the same, whereas others do not.[5,23] Others separate diagnostic errors from diagnosis depending on whether the error occurred during the diagnostic process versus the final outcome of the process.[24] Whether the definition of a diagnostic error should include unavoidable errors or if it stems solely from a failure in the diagnostic process is also a point of contention.[23,25]

Although several definitions have been proposed for diagnostic error, a distinct lack of consensus remains. Five major definitions of diagnostic error, described in later discussion, have emerged in the diagnostic error movement.

Graber and colleagues[26] define a diagnostic error as a diagnosis that was unintentionally delayed when sufficient information was available earlier, wrong if another diagnosis was made before the correct one, or missed based on eventual discovery of more definitive diagnostic information. Furthermore, they divide diagnostic errors into system-related if related to organizational barriers, cognitive when there is error in the clinician's reasoning, and no-fault errors. No-fault errors refer to errors that stem from factors outside of the clinician's or health system's control, such as extremely atypical disease presentation or delivery presentation of misleading information by the patient.[27]

Schiff and colleagues[25] define diagnostic errors as a mistake or failure in the diagnostic process leading to a misdiagnosis, missed diagnosis, or delayed diagnosis.

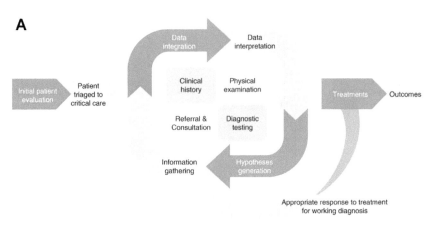

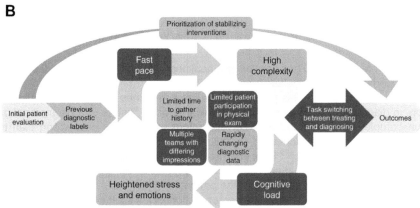

Fig. 2. (A) The ICU diagnostic process superimposed with (B) the common hindrances to diagnosing critically ill patients. (From Bergl P, Nanchal R, Singh H. Diagnostic Error in the Critically III: Defining the Problem and Exploring Next Steps to Advance Intensive Care Unit Safety. Annals of the American Thoracic Society. 15.8 (2018); with permission.)

They noted that not all errors in the diagnostic process will lead to a missed, delayed, or wrong diagnosis and that not all errors will result in patient harm.[24] In this model, diagnosis is an intermediate process-based outcome of the process of diagnosis, whereas a resultant adverse event would be a true patient-oriented outcome.[28]

Newman-Toker[23] distinguishes between diagnostic process failures and incorrect diagnostic labeling. Process failures occur when there is an error in the diagnostic workup. In contrast, diagnostic labeling failure occurs when the actual diagnosis the patient receives is incorrect. A preventable diagnostic error then occurs when a diagnostic process failure results in a diagnostic labeling failure.[23] Such an error is distinct from a near miss, which occurs when there is a mistake in the diagnostic process without a diagnostic labeling failure.[23]

Singh[9] uses the concept of missed opportunities to define diagnostic error. A missed opportunity suggests that something different could have been done in the diagnostic process to make the correct diagnosis sooner. In this framework, a diagnostic error occurs if there is unequivocal evidence of a missed opportunity during the diagnostic process to establish a timely and accurate diagnosis, regardless of whether harm occurred.[9] These missed opportunities may or may not be preventable and may or may not cause harm. In Singh's framework, there is a specific focus on preventable errors that cause harm as targets for intervention.

After evaluating these various definitions, the 2015 NAM report attempted to operationalize a cohesive definition of diagnostic error. It defined diagnostic errors as "failure to (a) establish an accurate and timely explanation of the patient's health problem(s) or (b) communicate that explanation to the patient."[2] This definition emphasizes the need for accurate and timely diagnosis, which is conceptually separated from a working diagnosis that may not be precise or complete. It also centers on the patient as the primary party at risk for harm from a diagnostic error. Furthermore, failure to communicate a diagnosis to the patient constitutes a diagnostic error. This definition allows for each component of the diagnostic process to be evaluated separately for measurement purposes.

MEASUREMENT

Although it is known that diagnostic errors continue to occur and cause harm, a primary reason for the lack of progress in this field has been the inability to accurately measure the incidence and impact of diagnostic errors.[2,29] Accurate measurement of diagnostic performance is widely acknowledged to be necessary for any systemic efforts to decrease diagnostic error, yet no universally accepted method of measuring diagnostic error currently exists.[29] The ICU is not immune to these difficulties in measuring diagnostic errors. Although the ICU is resource-rich in terms of rapid access to a wide variety of diagnostic modalities, efforts to advance measurement of diagnostic error among the critically ill face significant obstacles.[30] Here, the authors review the major systems of identifying and quantifying diagnostic error in the ICU.

Historically, autopsies have been the primary method of studying diagnostic errors in intensive care settings.[31] A review by Winters and colleagues[11] of 5863 autopsies found that 28% of autopsies reported at least 1 misdiagnosis, and a potentially fatal diagnostic error occurred in 8% of autopsies. Although autopsy allows for a comprehensive evaluation of select cases, the most obvious limitation is that an autopsy can only evaluate for diagnostic error when the outcome is death.[32] Also, because physicians and patient families are more likely to pursue autopsy if there is diagnostic uncertainty at time of death, this indication bias raises concern that rates of diagnostic error from autopsy may overestimate the true incidence of diagnostic error.[31] Nonetheless, autopsy remains an important source of information regarding diagnostic errors in select ICU patients, and future research efforts using autopsy to study targeted groups of ICU patients may provide useful information.[33–36]

Another approach to studying diagnostic errors has focused on medical malpractice claims.[17] Diagnostic errors are common among patients who file medical malpractice claims and tend to be the most costly and dangerous.[37] A large study analyzing 25 years' worth of malpractice data by Newman-Toker and colleagues[38] found that of the 350,706 paid claims, diagnostic errors were the leading type (28.6%) and accounted for the highest proportion of total payments (35.2%), with diagnostic errors that resulted in death or disability occurring almost twice as often as other error categories.[17] In addition, patients in the ICU were at significantly higher risk to experience a diagnostic error. Although providing large-scale data, malpractice claims-based data are inherently limited only to patients for whom a medical malpractice claim is filed. Thus, although it can provide insights into a specific subset of ICU patients, diagnostic error rates generated by claims analysis are inherently limited in their generalizability.

Another approach to quantifying diagnostic error in critical care has been surveys of critical care clinicians.[39] Surveys that have also been used to query critical care clinicians on their experiences with diagnostic errors have noted their presence and effect in the ICU, but such methods are inherently limited by the self-selection of respondents, and validation of the data collected in this manner is difficult.[38] Similarly, solicitation of self-reported diagnostic errors has determined the presence of diagnostic error in health care settings, such as the ICU, but is limited in its scope.[40,41] These limitations also extend to data from morbidity and mortality conferences in critical care. Although these data sources corroborate the widespread presence of diagnostic error in critical care, they cannot yield generalizable data or quantify the frequency of errors.[42,43]

The complicated and critical nature of patients in the ICU also makes them more prone to diagnostic errors during patient handoffs that occur between clinicians.[44] Data from surveys evaluating handoffs in critical care have noted that intensivists consider inadequate communication during handoff to be a significant cause of diagnostic errors.[45] Literature related to handoffs has focused primarily on the information contained in reports available in the electronic medical record and do not specifically evaluate for resultant diagnostic errors.[46]

In terms of determining generalizable rates of diagnostic error in the ICU, one of the primary barriers to measurement of diagnostic error has been the inability to evaluate large populations of critical care patients. Although the electronic medical record contains vast amounts of patient information, the volume of patient data within it is sometimes overwhelmingly large, particularly in ICU patients. Reviewing and analyzing these large volumes of data are challenging. Approaches designed to overcome such challenges have been developed. The Symptom-Disease Pair Analysis methodology is a technique to identify the likelihood of errors based on the diagnosis coded in large conglomerates of electronic health records, such as administrative data sets.[47] This method can be used for presentations of diseases with closely linked symptoms, such as emergency room visits for nonspecific dizziness followed by subsequent hospital admissions for cerebrovascular accidents within a short timeframe, by applying algorithms based on biologic plausibility combined with statistical analysis to determine the likelihood of an error in diagnosis. This allows for rapid evaluation of large data sets, but this approach relies on the presence of a specific outcome and does not allow for evaluation of individual patient charts in cases whereby a diagnostic error is suspected (eg, evaluation of the specific clinical circumstances in which the error occurred). Furthermore, it relies solely on the diagnoses coded for in the patient's electronic health record and thus may be insufficiently sensitive to detect diagnostic errors.

Finally, electronic triggers can be applied to large amounts of clinical data to detect diagnostic errors. The Safer Dx e-trigger tool framework can be used to develop electronic triggers to screen large sets of electronic health records to identify cohorts who may have experienced diagnostic errors, monitor event rates, and potentially identify patients at high risk for an adverse event in the future.[48] Examples of electronic triggers relevant to critical care might include unexpected transfers from the general medical floor to the ICU, initiation of inpatient rapid response team, or code event with death before discharge. For example, this type of triggering algorithm could aid in error identification for a patient with an emergent transfer from the general medical floor to the ICU who was found to have a pneumothorax that had been missed on a radiograph earlier during admission. Once flagged, however, charts identified by this method require comprehensive review to confirm the presence of a diagnostic error and often lack specificity for errors.

One approach to analyzing patient charts based off trigger events is the Safer Dx instrument, which contains a variety of questions designed to evaluate diagnostic processes and identify the presence or absence of diagnostic errors.[8] This instrument is based on the Safer Dx framework that assesses the structure, process, and outcome aspects of diagnosis in order to detect process breakdowns, which led to diagnostic errors. Although comprehensive in terms of record review, this methodology is limited in its ability to evaluate clinicians' cognitive processing or other information not documented in the patient chart. Nonetheless, it does provide a potential conceptual foundation for system-wide measurement of diagnostic error and has been applied in the ICU to study diagnostic error in critical care.[30]

A primary limitation of the aforementioned methodologies is that they are retrospective, which precludes the possibility of real-time intervention. Unfortunately, prospective methodology for real-time surveillance of diagnostic error remains in the development stage and is not currently used in active diagnostic errors research.[29] As measurement methods evolve, they should address concepts such as uncertainty and clinician calibration in order to optimize the balance between reducing overuse and addressing underuse of diagnostic tests and other resources.[29,49] Evolved methods will be essential for advancing diagnostic error research and prevention in critical care medicine.

RECOMMENDATIONS FROM 2015 NATIONAL ACADEMY OF MEDICINE REPORT

The 2015 report by the NAM on improving diagnosis in medicine remains a landmark publication in the patient safety movement. Despite recent advances, however, progress on the development of measurement instruments and interventions to reduce diagnostic error remains slow.[50] The report's authoring committee generated 8 key recommendations to improve diagnostic safety and decrease diagnostic error in health care, which are summarized in **Box 1**. They also emphasized that increasing diagnostic excellence is a moral, professional, and public health imperative, a call that continues to be corroborated by other prominent organizations.[2,11–14] Combating

---

Box 1
Key recommendations from the 2015 National Academy of Medicine report, *Improving Diagnosis in Healthcare*

1. Facilitate more effective teamwork in the diagnostic process among health care professionals, patients, and their families.

2. Enhance health care professional education and training in the diagnostic process.

3. Ensure health information technologies support patients and health care professional in the diagnostic process.

4. Develop and deploy approaches to identify, learn from, and reduce diagnostic errors and near misses in clinical practice.

5. Establish a work system and culture that supports the diagnostic process and improvements in diagnostic performance.

6. Develop a reporting environment and medical liability system that facilitates improved diagnosis by learning from diagnostic errors and near misses.

7. Design a payment and care delivery environment that supports the diagnostic process.

8. Provide dedicated funding for research on the diagnostic process and diagnostic errors.

Adapted from Box S-1. Goals for Improving Diagnosis and Reducing Diagnostic Error, National Academies of Sciences, Engineering, and Medicine, 2015. Improving Diagnosis in Health Care. Washington, DC: The National Academies Press; with permission.

the scourge of diagnostic error is especially relevant in critical care medicine, where the consequences of such errors are most likely to be life-altering or lethal.

SUMMARY

Despite the significant advances made by the patient safety movement to decrease preventable error, significant gaps remain in the understanding of diagnostic errors in critical care medicine. The complexity of the diagnostic process makes operationalizing a definition of diagnostic error and measurement of said error challenging, and these challenges have thus far precluded systemic efforts at preventing diagnostic errors in the ICU. There is, however, growing awareness of the danger posed by diagnostic errors as well as the need for targeted research on diagnostic errors.

CLINICS CARE POINTS

- Diagnostic error remains difficult to define and quantify.
- Diagnostic errors are present and cause harm in the intensive care unit.
- Diagnostic error remains understudied in critical care medicine and more research is needed.

DISCLOSURE

The authors have no conflicts of interest relevant to this article to disclose. No funding was secured for this article.

REFERENCES

1. IOM to err is human: building a safer health system. Washington, D.C: National Academy Press; 2000.
2. National Academies of Sciences, Engineering, and Medicine. Improving diagnosis in health care. Washington, DC: The National Academies Press; 2015.
3. Berner E. Diagnostic error in medicine: introduction. Adv Health Sci Educ Theory Pract 2009;14(suppl 1):1–5.
4. Graber M, Gordon R, Franklin N. Reducing diagnostic errors in medicine: what's the goal? Acad Med 2002;77(10):981–92.
5. Newman-Toker D, Pronovost P. Diagnostic errors – the next frontier for patient safety. J Am Med Assoc 2009;301:1060–2.
6. Thammasitboon S, Thammasitboon S, Singhal G. Diagnosing diagnostic error. Curr Probl Pediatr Adolesc Health Care 2013;43(9):227–31.
7. Graber M. The incidence of diagnostic error in medicine. BMJ Qual Saf 2013;22(Suppl 2):21–7.
8. Singh H, Sittig D. Advancing the science of measurement of diagnostic errors in healthcare: the safer Dx framework. BMJ Qual Saf 2015;24(2):727–31.
9. Singh H. Editorial: helping health care organizations to define diagnostic errors as missed opportunities in diagnosis. Joint Comm J Qual Patient Saf 2014;40(3):99–101.
10. Cresswell K, Panesar S, Salvilla S, et al. Global research priorities to better understand the burden of iatrogenic harm in primary care: an international Delphi exercise. PLoS Med 2013;10(11):e1001554.
11. Winters B, Custer J, Galvagno SM Jr, et al. Diagnostic errors in the intensive care unit: a systematic review of autopsy studies. BMJ Qual Saf 2012;21(11):894–902.

12. ECRI Institute. Top 10 patient safety concerns for healthcare organizations 2018. ECRI Institute; 2018. Available at: https://www.ecri.org/EmailResources/PSRQ/Top10/2018_PSTop10_ExecutiveBrief.pdf.
13. ECRI Institute. Top 10 patient safety concerns for healthcare organizations 2019. ECRI Institute; 2019. Available at: https://assets.ecri.org/PDF/White-Papers-and-Reports/2019-Top10-Patient-Safety-Concerns-Exec-Summary.pdf.
14. ECRI Institute. Top 10 patient safety concerns for healthcare organizations 2020. ECRI Institute; 2020. Available at: https://assets.ecri.org/PDF/White-Papers-and-Reports/2020-Top-10-Patient-Safety-Executive-Brief.pdf.
15. Anonymous Author. Diagnostic errors top ECRI Institute's patient safety concerns for 2018: new report examines root causes for serious patient safety events. J Health Care Compliance 2018;20(2):43–4.
16. Bergl P, Nanchal R, Singh H. Diagnostic error in the critically ill: defining the problem and exploring next steps to advance intensive care unit safety. Ann Am Thorac Soc 2018;15(8):903–7.
17. Saber-Tehrani A, Lee HW, Matthews S, et al. 25-year summary of US malpractice claims for diagnostic errors 1986–2010: an analysis from the National Practitioner Data Bank. BMJ Qual Saf 2013;22(8):672–80.
18. Garrouste Orgeas M, Timsit JF, Soufir L, et al. Impact of adverse events on outcomes in intensive care unit patients. Crit Care Med 2008;36(7):2041–7.
19. Rothschild JM, Landrigan CP, Cronin JW, et al. The Critical Care Safety Study: the incidence and nature of adverse events and serious medical errors in intensive care. Crit Care Med 2005;33(8):1694–700.
20. Valentin A, Capuzzo M, Guidet B, et al. Patient safety in intensive care: results from the multinational Sentinel Events Evaluation (SEE) study. Intensive Care Med 2006;32(10):1591–8.
21. Marquet K, Claes N, De Troy E, et al. One fourth of unplanned transfers to a higher level of care are associated with a highly preventable adverse event: a patient record review in six Belgian hospitals. Crit Care Med 2015;43(5):1053–61.
22. IOM. Patient safety: achieving a New Standard for care. Washington, District of Columbia: The National Academies Press; 2004.
23. Newman-Toker DE. A unified conceptual model for diagnostic errors: underdiagnosis, overdiagnosis, and misdiagnosis. Diagnosis (Berl) 2014;1(1):43–8.
24. Berenson R, Upadhyay DK, Kaye DR. Placing diagnosis errors on the policy agenda. Washington, DC: Urban Institute. Available at: www.urban.org/research/publication/placing-diagnosis-errors-policy-agenda. Accessed April 1, 2021.
25. Schiff GD, Hasan O, Kim S, et al. Diagnostic error in medicine: analysis of 583 physician-reported errors. Arch Intern Med 2009;169(20):1881–7.
26. Graber ML, Franklin N, Gordon R. Diagnostic error in internal medicine. Arch Intern Med 2005;165(13):1493–9.
27. Kassirer JP. Our stubborn quest for diagnostic certainty. A cause of excessive testing. N Engl J Med 1989;320(22):1489–91.
28. Schiff GD, Leape LL. Commentary: how can we make diagnosis safer? Acad Med 2012;87(2):135–8.
29. Singh H, Bradford A, Goeschel C. Operational measurement of diagnostic safety: state of the science. Diagnosis (Berl) 2020;8(1):51–65.
30. Bergl P, Taneja A, El-Kareh R, et al. 1321: frequency of diagnostic errors and related risk factors in the MICU: a retrospective cohort study. Crit Care Med 2019;47(1 Suppl 1):637.

31. Shojania KG, Burton EC, McDonald KM, et al. Changes in rates of autopsy-detected diagnostic errors over time: a systematic review. J Am Med Assoc 2003;289(21):2849–56.
32. Podbregar M, Voga G, Krivec B, et al. Should we confirm our clinical diagnostic certainty by autopsies? Intensive Care Med 2001;27(11):1750–5.
33. Tejerina E, Esteban A, Fernández-Segoviano P, et al. Clinical diagnoses and autopsy findings: discrepancies in critically ill patients*. Crit Care Med 2012;40(3):842–6.
34. Carmignani M, Valle G, Volpe AR. Shall we resuscitate autopsy in the intensive care unit? Crit Care Med 2012;40(3):1003–4.
35. Nadrous HF, Afessa B, Pfeifer EA, et al. The role of autopsy in the intensive care unit. Mayo Clin Proc 2003;78(8):947–50.
36. Silfvast T, Takkunen O, Kolho E, et al. Characteristics of discrepancies between clinical and autopsy diagnoses in the intensive care unit: a 5-year review. Intensive Care Med 2003;29(2):321–4.
37. Gupta A, Snyder A, Kachalia A, et al. Malpractice claims related to diagnostic errors in the hospital. BMJ Qual Saf 2018;27:53–60.
38. Newman-Toker DE, Schaffer AC, Yu-Moe CW, et al. Serious misdiagnosis-related harms in malpractice claims: the "Big Three" - vascular events, infections, and cancers [published correction appears in Diagnosis (Berl). 2020 May 16;8(1):127-128]. Diagnosis (Berl) 2019;6(3):227–40.
39. Kaur AP, Levinson AT, Monteiro JFG, et al. The impact of errors on healthcare professionals in the critical care setting. J Crit Care 2019;52:16–21.
40. Okafor N, Payne VL, Chathampally Y, et al. Using voluntary reports from physicians to learn from diagnostic errors in emergency medicine. Emerg Med J 2016;33(4):245–52. https://doi.org/10.1136/emermed-2014-204604.
41. Schiff GD. Minimizing diagnostic error: the importance of follow-up and feedback. Am J Med 2008;121:S38–42.
42. Cifra CL, Jones KL, Ascenzi J, et al. The morbidity and mortality conference as an adverse event surveillance tool in a paediatric intensive care unit. BMJ Qual Saf 2014;23(11):930-8. doi: 10.1136/bmjqs-2014-003000.
43. Cifra CL, Jones KL, Ascenzi JA, et al. Diagnostic errors in a PICU: insights from the morbidity and mortality conference. Pediatr Crit Care Med 2015;16(5):468–76.
44. Colvin MO, Eisen LA, Gong MN. Improving the patient handoff process in the intensive care unit: keys to reducing errors and improving outcomes. Semin Respir Crit Care Med 2016;37(1):96–106.
45. Lane-Fall M, Collard M, Turnbull A, et al. ICU attending handoff practices: results from a national survey of academic intensivists. Crit Care Med 2016;44(4):690–8.
46. Usher MG, Fanning C, Wu D, et al. Information handoff and outcomes of critically ill patients transferred between hospitals. J Crit Care 2016;36:240–5.
47. Liberman A, Newman-Toker D. Symptom-disease pair analysis of diagnostic error (SPADE): a conceptual framework and methodological approach for unearthing misdiagnosis-related harms using big data. BMJ Qual Saf 2018;27(7):557–66.
48. Bhise V, Sittig D, Vagahani V, et al. An electronic trigger based on care escalation to identify preventable adverse events in hospitalised patients. BMJ Qual Saf 2018;27(3):241–6.
49. Schiff GD, Martin SA, Eidelman DH, et al. Ten principles for more conservative, care-full diagnosis. Ann Intern Med 2018;169:643–5.
50. Hall KK, Shoemaker-Hunt S, Hoffman L, et al. Making healthcare safer III: a critical analysis of existing and emerging patient safety practices [Internet]. Rockville (MD): Agency for Healthcare Research and Quality (US); 2020. Diagnostic Errors.

Diagnostic Error in the Critically Ill: A Hidden Epidemic?

Paul A. Bergl, MD[a,b,]*, Yan Zhou, MD[c,d]

KEYWORDS

- Diagnostic error • Medical errors • Autopsy • Intensive care units • Patient safety
- Patient harm

KEY POINTS

- Fatal diagnostic errors occur in approximately 2% to 8% of patients who die in a modern intensive care unit (ICU); overall, major diagnostic errors are found in approximately 10% of critically ill adults and children.
- Diagnostic errors in the ICU usually do not originate from exotic or rare conditions. Instead, common cardiovascular disorders, such as myocardial infarction and pulmonary embolism, and common infectious syndromes, such as bacterial pneumonia, account for most major diagnostic errors among the critically ill.
- An individual patient's severity of illness, complexity, typicality or atypicality of their signs and symptoms, and immunocompetency all likely factor into their risk for experiencing a diagnostic error in the ICU. Systemic factors, such as ICU strain, may also increase the risk for errors.
- Diagnostic errors are the most devastating and costly types of errors that occur in hospitalized patients. In settled malpractice cases, more than 60% of patients who experience diagnostic errors suffered major permanent harms or death as consequences.

INTRODUCTION

Although no universal definition exists, the framework proposed by the National Academy of Medicine provides a systematic approach to understanding the epidemiology of diagnostic errors in the intensive care unit (ICU).[1] The National Academy of Medicine's framework recognizes the complicated nature of the diagnostic process. In the practice of critical care, this process includes upstream care (such as occurs in a hospital ward, emergency room, or operating theater), the various steps in obtaining

[a] Department of Critical Care, Gundersen Lutheran Medical Center, 1900 South Avenue, Mail Stop LM3-001, La Crosse, WI 54601, USA; [b] Department of Medicine, University of Wisconsin School of Medicine and Public Health, Madison, WI, USA; [c] Department of Critical Care Medicine, Geisinger Medical Center, 100 N Academy Avenue, Danville, PA 17822, USA; [d] Geisinger Commonwealth School of Medicine, Scranton, PA, USA
* Corresponding author.
E-mail address: pabergl@gundersenhealth.org

Crit Care Clin 38 (2022) 11–25
https://doi.org/10.1016/j.ccc.2021.09.005
0749-0704/22/© 2021 Elsevier Inc. All rights reserved.

criticalcare.theclinics.com

and interpreting additional diagnostic data, and the timely provision of accurate diagnostic hypotheses that are effectively communicated to the patient or surrogates.[1]

However, given the relatively recent origin of these frameworks, the understanding of diagnostic error in the ICU must encompass other approaches to identifying and measuring such errors. In this chapter, the authors first delve into the epidemiologic data provided by autopsies, the historical "gold standard" for identifying diagnostic errors. Next, they examine epidemiologic data from other methods of measuring diagnostic errors in the ICU. Because the number of contemporary ICU-oriented studies of diagnostic errors are limited, the authors also examine broader trends in misdiagnosis among other high-acuity patient populations and finally review diagnostic error-related risk factors and outcomes in critically ill patients.

AUTOPSIES AND THE EPIDEMIOLOGY OF DIAGNOSTIC ERRORS AMONG THE CRITICALLY ILL
A Brief History

For centuries, physicians have sought to learn from patients' deaths and to calibrate their diagnostic accuracy. As early as the third century BC, postmortem dissections helped inform our understanding of human anatomy and the broader human condition.[2] But it was not until the eighteenth century AD that luminaries such as Herman Boerhaave and Marie François Xavier Bichat began to promulgate the autopsy as a tool for enhancing clinical diagnostic accuracy.[2] Building from these traditions, Sir William Osler arguably developed the modern framework for diagnostic error by refining his diagnostic acumen through postmortem examination of his own patients.[3] By the early twentieth century, autopsy ascended to the gold standard for settling the uncertainty of antemortem diagnosis.

Within this historical context, autopsies have proved one of the best approaches to identifying diagnostic errors. Indeed, one of the first published compendia of diagnostic errors appeared in the literature over 100 years ago. In his 1912 review of 3000 autopsies, Cabot cataloged common diagnostic pitfalls and quantified the frequency of diagnostic "correctness" for various diagnoses (with clinicians of Cabot's era missing hepatic abscesses and acute pericarditis nearly always).[4] Subsequently, Goldman and colleagues cemented the value of modern autopsy in 3 eras spanning 1960 to 1980.[5] In this seminal study, Goldman and colleagues found that nearly 10% of autopsies revealed a major error that could have potentially contributed to the patient's death. Despite rapidly advancing diagnostic technology, rates of major misdiagnoses remained stable in all 3 studied decades.

Persistent errors in modern medicine revealed by autopsy
In the 1980s and 1990s, the published literature blossomed with autopsy-based cohort studies examining premortem and postmortem diagnostic discrepancies.[6] Shojania and colleagues[6] conducted a systematic review of published autopsy cohorts from 1966 through 2002, which identified 53 distinct cohorts that included more than 10,000 autopsied patients. The investigators found a statistically significant decrease in major diagnostic errors toward the end of the twentieth century; nonetheless, even in the early 2000s, lethal misdiagnoses still accounted for an estimated 35,000 deaths annually in US hospitals.

This early work by Goldman and subsequent systematic review by Shojania ultimately proved prescient. In large cohorts from the twenty-first century, potentially lethal misdiagnoses continue to be found in approximately 10% of autopsied patients.[7,8] Further, major diagnostic discrepancies still occur in nearly 1 in 5 autopsied patients who die in the hospital.[7-9] Most concerning, despite significant reductions in the rates of diagnostic discrepancies in the twentieth century, these improvements seem to be leveling off recently.[6,7,9]

Limitations of extrapolating "error rates" from autopsy studies
Before delving into additional lessons from autopsy data, one must consider the inherent limitations of using nonrepresentative samples of deceased patients and reporting "error rates" based on these samples. In the review by Shojania and colleagues, the median autopsy rate was 37%.[6] For ease of math, consider a large hypothetical cohort of 10,000 patients in which 33% of deceased patients undergo autopsy and in which major diagnostic errors are found in 10% of these autopsies. In this hypothetical cohort, errors would be found in only 333 patients (10% of the 3333 patients who were autopsied) or only 3.3% of patients. Assuming that autopsied patients are selected due to specific factors, such as diagnostic uncertainty or younger age, it is possible that there were few to no major errors in the remaining 67% of deceased patients who were not autopsied. In this hypothetical cohort, the probability of error occurring is thus 3.3%.

Recognizing the referral bias for autopsy, the investigators of meta-analyses of autopsy cohorts have sought to use linear or nonlinear models to account for these limitations and to extrapolate a theoretic error rate in a population of decedents who all undergo autopsy.[6,10] For example, Shojania and colleagues calculated that major diagnostic errors would be identified in 8% to 24% of autopsies even at a hypothetical autopsy rate of 100%. This estimate is supported by the finding that major error rates were 8% even in cohorts in which 80% or more of decedents were autopsied.[6]

A system for judging errors
Goldman's seminal publication on diagnostic discrepancies at autopsy also established a modern scheme for classifying such discrepancies. An explanation of the Goldman system is shown in **Table 1**. Since Goldman's initial descriptions of these classes, the investigators have often used slight modifications with tailored verbiage.[7,11,12] However, almost any modern autopsy cohort appearing in the

Table 1
Overview of Goldman classifications of diagnostic error found on autopsy

Major discrepancies or misdiagnoses	
Class I	Major diagnostic discrepancies likely contributed to the patient's death. Knowledge of the correct diagnosis before death would have led to changes in management that could have prolonged survival.
Class II	Major discrepancies were present, but detection of the error before death would not have changed survival. Missed diagnoses did not contribute to the patient's death.
Minor discrepancies	
Class III	Minor diagnoses that were not directly related to the cause of death. Symptoms of the diagnosis were present before death and should have been treated. Alternatively, the diagnosis may have been asymptomatic but would have eventually affected prognosis.
Class IV	Minor occult diagnoses that were not diagnosable before death. These diagnoses had no relation to the cause of death and may not have even caused symptoms but may have possible epidemiologic or genetic importance (eg, incidentally identified and asymptomatic carcinoma in situ).

literature will use some version of this classification system. Class I and II discrepancies are considered "major" errors and are most commonly the primary outcome of interest in published cohorts.

Trends in major misdiagnoses in autopsied intensive care unit patients

Although several published cohorts were restricted to autopsies performed on ICU patients, the 2002 meta-analysis by Shojania and colleagues was the first to identify that ICU (vs non-ICU) patients might be at increased risk for major errors. Their meta-analysis demonstrated that major misdiagnoses were significantly more common among ICU decedents (odds ratio 2.12, 95% confidence interval 1.42–3.16).[6] These findings, however, were subsequently repudiated by a large cohort study of autopsied patients in Berlin, Germany that spanned 2 decades from 1988 to 2008.[7] In this analysis of 1800 cases, the investigators found that rates of major discrepancies were equally common among ICU and non-ICU decedents.[7] To directly compare rates of major discrepancies between the ICU and non-ICU populations, however, would require both an identical autopsy rate in each group *and* an identical base rate of errors in these 2 groups; from 1988 to 2008, the percentage of autopsies coming from ICU patients ranged from 25% to 67%. As such, these comparative studies cannot accurately determine whether ICU patients are at higher risk for major discrepancies than other hospitalized patients.

Fortunately, myriad studies have specifically examined ICU patients who undergo autopsy, and these studies provide compelling data that rates of diagnostic discrepancy among the critically ill are similar to rates among all inpatients. In 2012, Winters and colleagues conducted a focused systematic review and meta-analysis of diagnostic errors in the ICU.[10] They identified 31 separate cohorts spanning the years 1988 through 2011 and described the outcomes of 5863 decedents from these cohorts. Perhaps unsurprisingly, the investigators noted that 8% of autopsies on ICU patients identified a Goldman Class I error[10]—a hauntingly familiar frequency that echoed the trends in the broader autopsy literature. An additional 15% of patients had class II errors; thus, about 1 in 4 autopsied ICU patients died with a major missed diagnosis or misdiagnosis.

More recent analyses of autopsied patients have provided conflicting data on whether diagnostic accuracy may be improving in the twenty-first century ICU. In one cohort at a major teaching hospital in Dublin, Ireland in which 32% of deceased patients were autopsied, fewer than 8% of autopsied ICU patients had a Goldman class I or class II diagnostic error.[13] Although the investigators posited that technological advances have augmented diagnostic accuracy, their use of a stringent definition of Goldman class I errors may account for fewer errors adjudicated. To qualify as a class I error, all of the following conditions needed to be present: (1) accurate diagnosis was possible premortem; (2) the condition was unlikely to have occurred while the patient was already moribund; (3) there was effective treatment available for the missed diagnosis, there were no contraindications to the treatment, and the treatment could have been introduced early enough to affect the patient's outcome; and (4) the patient must not have refused evaluation or treatment.[13] These stricter criteria deviate from traditional interpretations of the Goldman systems[11] but also may better reflect the dynamic and time-sensitive nature of critical care. Further, in this cohort, autopsied patients were significantly younger and had significantly shorter ICU lengths of stay[13]; these findings lend additional evidence for referral bias in autopsy studies.

A separate study in a major Belgian teaching hospital found that rates of major premortem/postmortem discrepancies in ICU patients between 2016 and 2018 were only 2.3% for Goldman class I and 7.8% for Goldman class II misclassifications.[14] Notably, approximately half of ICU decedents were autopsied, a rate that greatly exceeds typical autopsy rates in the twentieth century.[15] Also noteworthy was that autopsy rates and frequencies of major discrepancies were stable when compared with previously published cohorts from 2004 and 2007 at the same institution.[16,17] A similar cohort from Finland, which was also published since Winters' meta-analysis and also had an autopsy rate approaching 50%, found class I and II errors in fewer than 10% of ICU patients.[18] Together, these studies with high autopsy rates may attenuate some referral bias seen in other autopsy cohorts, but younger patients in the Finnish cohort were still significantly more likely to be autopsied.[18]

On the other hand, Tejerina and colleagues published a similarly sized retrospective cohort study of autopsied ICU patients in 2018.[19] The investigators found that rates of Goldman class I errors among autopsied patients persisted at 8.4%.[19] In this study, autopsy was performed on 215 (32%) of 671 adults who had died in a mixed medical-surgical ICU in Madrid, Spain. Despite the aforementioned Belgian and Finnish studies from the past decade suggesting a favorable trend,[14,18] Tejerina and colleagues demonstrated that major diagnostic errors in the modern ICU continue to arise frequently enough to merit our collective attention. Results from these studies are summarized and compared with data from Winters's meta-analysis in **Table 2**.

Trends among critically ill pediatric patients

Two recent systematic reviews have sought to estimate the incidence of major diagnostic errors in the pediatric intensive care unit (PICU).[20,21] In pooling 7 autopsy cohorts that were published between 1993 and 2011, Custer and colleagues derived a cohort of 498 PICU decedents.[20] Of these patients, 20% had experienced a major diagnostic error, with 6% being Goldman class I discrepancies. Cifra and colleagues[21] reviewed an additional 3 retrospective cohorts from 2014 and 2017; all cohorts were from single centers and found rates of major diagnostic error ranging from 6% to 54%. As elaborated later, the major outlier in this group was a cohort of pediatric patients who died on or shortly after receiving extracorporeal membrane oxygenator support (ECMO). After excluding this cohort, rates of major discrepancies (6%–23%) approximated broader trends from the adult autopsy literature.

Because of smaller number of clinical studies of pediatric patients, it is not clear whether rates of major discrepancies are decreasing among critically ill PICU and neonatal ICU (NICU) patients. The 2 most recent studies of PICU patients, which unfortunately contain small sample sizes of 39 and 99 patients, have found major discrepancies in only 6% to 12% of decedents.[22,23] Although these rates are among the lowest reported in any autopsy cohort of critically ill adults or children, the investigators in one of these studies openly acknowledged the inherent difficulties in using the Goldman classification system.[23] Citing the challenges in retrospectively determining how various comorbidities and multiple acute problems intersected to ultimately affect patient outcomes, these investigators suggest that their discrepancy rate may be an underestimate.[23]

Custer and colleagues also examined 6 cohorts of NICU patients, which included a robust sample of 1259 autopsied neonates when the cohorts were pooled.[20] After excluding an outlier cohort from India, major discrepancies were found in 1% to 7% (class I) and 14% to 57% (class II) of neonatal deaths. As Winters and colleagues[10] had described in their meta-analysis, Custer and colleagues found declining rates of major discrepancies in PICU and NICU cohorts with higher autopsy rates. Unfortunately, Custer and colleagues lacked a sufficient sample to estimate the expected rate of NICU and PICU errors at a theoretic autopsy rate of 100%.

Table 2 Summary of autopsy cohorts of critically ill adults			
Author and Publication Year	Total Number of Patients	Autopsy Rate	Rate of Goldman Class I Errors
Winters et al,[10] 2012	5863	43% (median for 31 studies)	8%
Fröhlich et al,[13] 2014	629	32.4%	2.4%
Liisanantti et al,[18] 2015	577	42.9%	4.4%
Tejerina et al,[19] 2018	671	32.0%	8.4%
Rusu et al,[14] 2021	888	53.2% (with 92.3% of autopsies reviewed for discrepancies)	2.3%

Diseases and concomitant diagnoses frequently found on autopsy

Beyond establishing approximate rates of diagnostic errors in the ICU, autopsy studies also illuminate diagnoses that intensivists are most likely to miss. Unsurprisingly, due to their sheer frequency, common diseases such as pulmonary embolism (PE), myocardial infarction, and infectious syndromes such as pneumonia account for the greatest number of Goldman class 1 discrepancies among adults,[9] including among the critically ill.[10] (To clarify this phenomenon, consider this hypothetical exercise in which 1% of fatal PE are missed antemortem and 50% of fatal cases of mucormycosis are also missed. Suppose that PE accounts for approximately 1000 deaths for every 100,000 deaths and mucormycosis causes 10 deaths for every 100,000 deaths. In a hypothetical population of 100,000 deceased patients, missed fatal PE will have caused 10 deaths, ie, 1% of the 1000 PE-associated deaths. However, missed fatal cases of mucormycosis will only have caused 5 deaths, ie, 50% of 10 mucormycosis-associated deaths. Thus, common diseases such as PE are generally more likely to be involved in errors, even if they are infrequently missed.) However, despite their relative rarity, major cardiovascular syndromes such as aortic dissection and cardiac tamponade, which are rapidly fatal but perhaps easily missed at bedside, are also among the most frequent class 1 errors identified in autopsied adults.[10] Intraabdominal catastrophes, such as ruptured aortic aneurysm, intraabdominal bleed, bowel infarction, pancreatitis, and perforated viscera, round out the remaining major diagnoses missed.[10] Among class 2 discrepancies, missed cancers are nearly as common as pulmonary embolism and myocardial infarction,[10] but their contributions to patients' deaths in the ICU are obviously less certain.

With respect to children, infections and cardiovascular events also predominate the class 1 discrepancies,[20,21] but neurologic diagnoses are nearly as common.[21] Further, congenital, metabolic, and genetic disorders, which are inherently unique to this population, comprise up to one-third of major discrepancies found in deceased critically ill children.[21] Among neonates, a variety of disorders had been missed antemortem and included a relatively even mix of missed bacterial and fungal infections, congenital malformations, genetic or metabolic disorders, central nervous system disease, and vascular events.[20]

In diagnostic discrepancy that involves missed infections, one important message has emerged from autopsy studies that merits special mention: invasive aspergillosis is often missed and deadly. In fact, Winters and colleagues found it to be one of the top 4 fatal misdiagnoses in adults, eclipsed only by pulmonary embolism, myocardial infarction, and pneumonia.[10] Aspergillosis seems to be the most frequently identified invasive fungal pathogen at autopsy,[24] and it is estimated that nearly half of the cases are missed antemortem.[25] In a study specifically reviewing ICU patients who had invasive aspergillosis diagnosed on postmortem examination, Tejerina and colleagues found that only 40% of these patients were clinically suspected of having the diagnosis before death even though nearly all patients had multiple risk factors.[26]

Autopsy studies of subpopulations of intensive care unit patients
Certain subpopulations of critically ill patients seem especially vulnerable to major diagnostic discrepancies. A concerning rate of diagnostic errors have been identified among pediatric patients who die while or after receiving ECMO.[27] In one hospital, 28% of deceased ECMO patients underwent autopsy and nearly 40% had class 1 discrepancies.[27] Myocardial infarction, unsuspected surgical complications, and adrenal hemorrhage were most commonly missed. In a study of adult recipients of hematopoetic stem cell transplantation, approximately 1 in 6 patients who underwent autopsy had a Goldman class I misdiagnosis attributed to missed infection.[28] Other studies affirm that diagnostic errors affect at least 20% of ICU patients who have a history of solid organ or bone marrow transplantation.[29,30] Cytomegalovirus, adenovirus, *Candida* species, and *Aspergillus* species accounted for the greatest proportion of missed antemortem infections.[28–30] Other patients with cancer seem to have a similarly elevated risk of error,[31,32] with invasive aspergillosis, pulmonary embolism, and cancer recurrence representing the prevailing major discrepancies.

Even among patients with a correct premortem primary diagnosis or seemingly obvious primary indication for ICU admission, major secondary diagnoses or concomitant diseases are also frequently missed. For example, among adjudicated cases of clinically suspected sepsis, Driessen and colleagues found that 13% of correctly diagnosed septic patients who died within 48 hours of ICU admission had other class 1 discrepancies, which included myocardial infarction, ruptured abdominal aortic aneurysm, and intraabdominal bleeding.[33] Studies of deceased patients in dedicated burn units also lend credence to the argument that fatal complications are often missed in patients who seemingly have an unambiguous primary diagnosis. In this population, fatal major diagnoses that might be potentially missed include pneumonia, intracerebral hemorrhage, myocardial infarction, and bowel infarction.[34,35]

Autopsy as diagnostic auditing tool
In addition to targeting specific populations, autopsy cohorts may be useful for adjudicating ICU diagnoses that are difficult to diagnose clinically, such ventilator-associated pneumonia (VAP). For example, Tejerina and colleagues evaluated a series of 253 ICU decedents' autopsies to determine the accuracy of the clinical diagnosis of VAP.[36] All patients had received greater than 48 hours of mechanical ventilation. Although autopsies included histologic evidence of pneumonia in 142 (56%) of patients, fewer than half of these patients had met clinical criteria for VAP before death. In this cohort, 3 definitions or sets of clinical criteria were used including the Clinical Pulmonary Infection Score and a combination of objective findings (leukocytosis, fever, purulent respiratory secretions, and radiographic infiltrate). Such disease-specific autopsy studies can provide benchmarking for accuracy of antemortem clinical diagnoses.

Autopsy summary
In summary, lethal missed diagnoses or misdiagnoses (Goldman class I) affect approximately 2% to 10% of autopsied ICU patients. Rates of error have remained largely stable since the 1960s although the most contemporary autopsy cohorts from the past decade suggest some improvement. To circumvent the inherent referral

bias in autopsy studies, experts have used mathematical models (based on a hypothetical 100% autopsy rate) to estimate an incidence of 6.3% for Goldman class 1 in deceased adult ICU patients[10] and a similar frequency among all patients who die in the hospital.[6] Further, based on autopsy meta-analyses, reasonable estimates suggest that between 30,000 and 40,000 of ICU patients die in part from lethal misdiagnoses.[6,10] Cardiovascular disorder and infections comprise the broad disease categories with the greatest number of class 1 errors; unexpected cancers account for a large proportion of class 2 errors. Based on autopsy studies, certain subpopulations of critically ill patients, particularly those with cancer or immunocompromising conditions, remain especially vulnerable to major misdiagnoses.

ESTIMATING THE FREQUENCY OF DIAGNOSTIC ERROR IN THE INTENSIVE CARE UNIT USING OTHER METHODS

Although autopsy is considered the gold standard for diagnostic accuracy, it has inherent limitations. First, these studies obviously only include patients who died; survivors of critical illness obviously may still experience diagnostic errors. Second, autopsy is typically performed in the context of diagnostic uncertainty and thus may not be representative of all ICU patients. Moreover, pathologists are generally applying the Goldman classification system to determine if discrepancies are present. Although the Goldman system provides definitions for classes of discrepancies, it does not provide a systematic framework for analyzing case records for errors. Further, it relies on the judgment of pathologists, who, although rigorously trained in their discipline, may not view diagnostic decision-making through the same lens as the bedside intensivist. Finally, the Goldman classification system does not delineate how the diagnostic process failed. Thus, alternative methods to adjudicating errors are necessary to better understand the scope of the epidemic of diagnostic error in the ICU.

Until recently, rigorous studies using alternative approaches to identifying diagnostic errors were lacking. The seminal Harvard Medical Practice Study published in 1991 pioneered the use of retrospective chart review to identify adverse events in hospitalized patients.[37] Although the Harvard study examined an array of medical errors, a noteworthy and often overlooked footnote is that this study was also one of the first studies to quantify the frequency and consequences of "diagnostic mishaps," which the investigators defined as "injuries that resulted from an improper or delayed diagnosis."[37] They found that diagnostic mishaps accounted for 7% to 14% of adverse events in hospitalized patients; among these diagnostic mishaps, care was deemed in negligent in 75% of cases.[37]

Since the Harvard study, other investigators have used similar methodology—that is, clinician-led retrospective chart review—to identify adverse events among critically ill patients.[38–40] As the Harvard study, these studies do not exclusively focus on diagnostic errors and have used a relatively simple definition for diagnostic failures. Nonetheless, they provide additional insight on the frequency of nonfatal diagnostic errors among critically ill patients. Physicians and nurses at the University College London Hospitals NHS Trust, a 700+ bed teaching hospital, reviewed ICU admissions from the general ward and found that 14% of these patients had experienced nonrecognition of a problem that was "clearly apparent" from physiologic or laboratory data.[38] A separate study reviewing admissions to 8 ICUs at 4 teaching hospitals found that diagnostic errors comprised 9% of iatrogenic events requiring critical care.[39] Finally, a study of ICU admissions among hospitalized patients in 6 Belgian acute care hospitals found that diagnostic errors occurred in 12% of adverse events leading to ICU admission.[40] Rates of diagnostic error from these studies, however, cannot be used to identify a true incidence, as the denominators are restricted to subsets of ICU patients. Thus, these studies would suggest that diagnostic errors are far less common when considering an entire population of critically ill patients.

A more precise approach to measuring diagnostic errors through retrospective review would involve unselected case records and a more rigorous review process focused exclusively on diagnosis. Several studies have applied the Safer Dx instrument to retrospectively ascertain whether diagnostic errors were present in ICU patients.[41-43] Developed by Singh and colleagues, this instrument requires trained reviewers to perform detailed analysis of the medical record by answering a series of prompts about the diagnostic process and decision-making.[44,45] These prompts force reviewers to unpack and deconstruct the case, an approach that may reduce the subjectivity of error determination.[45] This method has been shown to have strong test performance characteristics and reliability for finding diagnostic errors.[41,46] Further, it is enhanced by a robust framework centered on the diagnostic process[41] that other studies lack.[38-40]

Among the 3 studies using the Safer Dx approach, 2 evaluated PICU patients, and 1 evaluated adult medical ICU patients.[41-43] All 3 studies were limited to a single center. Davalos and colleagues focused their reviews on high-risk PICU patients, which they defined as those who underwent autopsy, had a recent outpatient health care visit, or were unexpectedly transferred from an acute care ward.[41] In their entire population of 214 pediatric patients, they identified diagnostic errors in 12.1% of cases. However, when restricting their analysis to patients who unexpectedly decompensated and subsequently required vasoactive medications or invasive mechanical ventilation within 24 hours, they found that nearly 30% of these patients had experienced errors. In a random, nonsequential cohort of 256 adults admitted to a medical ICU, errors were present in 7% of ICU patients, and only one-third of these errors were recognized in the first 24 hours of ICU care.[42] Finally, in a pilot study of 50 pediatric patients, Cifra and colleagues found that 8% of patients experienced a diagnostic error within the first 12 hours of PICU admission.[43] Together, these studies affirm that nonfatal diagnostic errors are relatively common. Further, they corroborate findings from autopsy studies that the incidence of diagnostic error depends on the specific subpopulations of ICU patients studied.

BROADER EPIDEMIOLOGIC TRENDS IN DIAGNOSTIC ERROR

Nearly all studies of diagnostic errors among the critically ill suffer from their limitation to certain subpopulations (ie, those undergoing autopsy, those experiencing deterioration on a general ward, and so forth). Thus, a true incidence of diagnostic errors among ICU patients remains largely unknown. A methodologically rigorous systematic review and meta-analysis by Gunderson and colleagues in 2020, however, likely establishes a reasonable lower limit.[47] Gunderson and colleagues aggregated data from 22 studies that included 80,026 hospitalized patients and found that only 0.7% of hospitalized patients experienced harmful diagnostic errors.[47] Because the investigators restricted their analyses to cases in which harm was present and directly caused by the error, and because these errors occurred largely outside of ICUs, this meta-analysis likely underestimates the true incidence for critically ill populations.

An alternative approach would be to measure disease-specific rates of diagnostic error. In a recent systematic review, Newman-Toker and colleagues sought to estimate national incidence of common diagnostic error categories.[48] Dubbed the "big three," these categories include infectious syndromes, cardiovascular events, and cancers and had previously been found to account for the most frequent and harmful errors in settled malpractice claims.[49] Although focused on broader epidemiologic trends, this study presents 2 key findings for the practicing intensivist. First, this study corroborates that diagnostic errors in the "big three" categories occur with alarming frequency; diagnostic error rates for aortic dissection, meningitis, spinal abscess, endocarditis, and arterial thromboembolism all exceed 20%.[48] Further, as one would expect intuitively, certain "big three" conditions prove particularly devastating when misdiagnosed or missed outright: most of the diagnostic errors in cardiovascular events and infectious syndromes—including the broad category of sepsis—result in major morbidity or death.[48]

Finally, there are paucity of studies examining the morbidity and financial harms that result from missed, delayed, or incorrect diagnoses in the ICU. Prospective studies of patients admitted to the hospital through an emergency department affirm that diagnostic errors have significant consequences, such as increased in-hospital mortality and longer length of stay.[50,51] Although settled malpractice claims are a nonrepresentative sample, they also represent a rich data source for quantifying such harm and identifying the specific disorders that, when missed or misdiagnosed, cause direct harm. As a group, malpractice claims for diagnostic failures, such as delayed diagnoses or misdiagnoses, account for the greatest share of disability and death[52] even though they are only the third most common cause for a malpractice claim (after surgical claims and medical treatment claims).[49] Over a 25-year period from 1986 to 2010, Saber Tehrani and colleagues found that the proportion of diagnostic error malpractice claims and payments had decreased about 50%, however.[52] Nonetheless, the mean per-claim payout in the United States for diagnostic errors was an inflation-adjusted $386,849 (US dollars),[52] and approximately two-thirds to three-quarters of filed claims entailed long-term disability or death.[49,52] The aforementioned "big three" categories of vascular events, infections, and cancers account for 74% of closed claims.[49]

RISK FACTORS POSITED OR KNOWN TO BE ASSOCIATED WITH DIAGNOSTIC ERRORS IN THE INTENSIVE CARE UNIT

Autopsy studies typically lack granular demographic and physiologic data from patients' ICU stays, so they cannot reliably identify specific patient risk factors for diagnostic errors.[12] Although other retrospective studies have included expanded patient-level data, they are limited by small sample sizes. Thus, this literature yields few consistent trends in risk factors for diagnostic error among critically ill patients.

Severity of Illness and Complexity

There are no autopsy studies that have quantified the risk of diagnostic error based on granular data on patient acuity. However, in the aforementioned retrospective ICU studies that used the Safer Dx instrument, severity of illness seemed to be a potential risk factor or marker of diagnostic errors. As noted in the study by Davalos, diagnostic errors were most common among patients who unexpectedly transferred to the ICU and subsequently received intensive care interventions (vasoactive medications, mechanical ventilation).[41] This finding suggests that ongoing deterioration may reflect a "diagnostic error in progress." Similarly, in their study of adult ICU patients, Bergl and colleagues found that severity of illness (based on the quick Sequential Organ Failure Assessment or qSOFA score) was independently and strongly associated with risk of diagnostic error in multivariate logistic regression analysis.[42]

Based on contemporary understanding of cognitive science, patient complexity has incredible face validity as a contributor to diagnostic error in the ICU. Unfortunately, there are no studies that have directly investigated the influence of patient complexity on diagnostic errors in the ICU setting. A whole body of literature strongly suggests that both biomedical complexity (eg, acuity of illness, burden of comorbidities) and contextual complexity (eg, patient-specific factors such as health literacy) increase the risk for medical errors.[53–55]

Typicality or Atypicality of Disease Presentation

Atypical presentations, vague complaints, and syndromes with highly variable symptoms all increase the risk for diagnostic error and its associated harms. Syndromes such as sepsis are already susceptible to inconsistency in diagnosis.[56] Not surprisingly, when patients with septic shock manifest vague symptoms, they experience significant diagnostic and therapeutic delays as compared with patients who have more explicit, localizable symptoms attributable to infection.[57] Similarly, patients with nonspecific chief complaints that are admitted to the hospital through the emergency room experience longer lengths of stay,[50] a complication that is likely attributable to diagnostic imprecision.

Immunocompromising Conditions

As discussed earlier, rates of diagnostic errors seem to be higher among critically ill patients who have cancer or have undergone solid-organ or hematological transplantation.[28,31,32] However, there are no studies directly comparing these populations with unselected ICU patients.

Recent Healthcare Before Index Intensive Care Unit Admission

Recent encounters with health care do not protect critically ill patients from diagnostic error. Intensivists must maintain especially high vigilance among ICU patients who recently had an emergency room visit. In patients with unscheduled return visits to the emergency department (ED) who subsequently are admitted to the ICU, the rate of diagnostic error in the index ED visit may exceed 40%.[58] Intensivists may also encounter patients recently discharged from the hospital and should recognize that patients may be readmitted due to diagnostic failure in the index admission as well. Rates of error in these populations, however, seem to reflect broader trends.[59]

Patient Risk Factors with Unclear or Unknown Effects on Diagnostic Error

No other clear trends have emerged from autopsy cohorts or other retrospective studies. Although nighttime admissions might be associated with more frequent errors in the PICU,[43] a study of adult ICU patients found no relationship between the time of ICU admission and error rates among adults.[42] The source of ICU admission (ward vs emergency room, for example) or specialty responsible for ICU care does not seem be consistently associated with errors.[13,41–43] Although one might expect that patients who die within 24 hours of ICU admission are more likely to have experienced error (which led to their rapid demise), studies have failed to show a statistically significant association.[14,20,42,60] Female sex has been implicated as a potential risk factor,[42] but this association is not consistent.[7,14] Admission to a community-based ICU, as opposed to an academic hospital, may be associated with a greater risk for error[7] but remains understudied.

Systemic Factors

Although difficult to study in actual clinical scenarios, limited time also likely increases the risk of error. In controlled experiments, time pressure clearly reduces diagnostic accuracy, mostly through the stress added to the task and the limits time imposes on generating a set of plausible hypotheses.[61] Ethnographic studies of inpatient teams have also identified time pressures as an impediment to sound diagnostic reasoning.[62] ICU and hospital strain have been posited as factors that increase the risk of medical errors and diminished quality of care,[63,64] but none of the descriptive studies of ICU errors have captured whether ICU capacity, strain, or time spent per patient affects diagnostic accuracy.

SUMMARY

Diagnostic error remains common in critical care despite advances in diagnostic testing and an increasing focus on patient safety and quality. Mortality from diagnostic errors is unacceptably high; at least 5% of deaths in the ICU are the consequence of fatal misdiagnosis. Clinicians most often misdiagnose or miss common diseases, such as cardiovascular events and infections, rather than rare conditions. Higher acuity of illness, complexity, (a)typicality of disease presentation, and immunocompromised status may represent patient-related risk factors for diagnostic error. Beyond mortality, diagnostic errors in the ICU likely cause significant morbidity and likely place an immense financial burden on the health care system.

CLINICS CARE POINTS

- Autopsies performed on critically ill patients frequently yield unanticipated findings, including major discrepancies that may have contributed to patients' deaths. This yield only declines slightly with increased rates of autopsy; thus, intensivists should pursue autopsy as a practice improvement strategy when technically and economically feasible.

- Intensivists should focus error-reduction efforts on cardiovascular events and infections, which are among the most common and most harmful categories of errors among the critically ill.

- Moreover, clinicians should conduct intensive diagnostic evaluations for the highest acuity patients and those with the most vague or atypical complaints as these patients appear particularly vulnerable to suffering morbidity and mortality from diagnostic errors.

DISCLOSURES

Drs P. Bergl and Y. Zhou have no disclosure or conflict of interest.

REFERENCES

1. Balogh EP, Miller BT, Ball JR, editors. Improving diagnosis in health care. Washington, DC: National Academies Press (US); 2015.
2. King LS, Meehan MC. A history of the autopsy. A review. Am J Pathol 1973;73(2):514–44.
3. Rodin AE. Osler's autopsies: their nature and utilization. Med Hist 1973;17(1):37–48.
4. Cabot RC. Diagnostic pitfalls identified during a study of three thousand autopsies. J Am Med Assoc 1912;LIX(26):2295–8.
5. Goldman L, Sayson R, Robbins S, et al. The value of the autopsy in three medical eras. N Engl J Med 1983;308(17):1000–5.
6. Shojania KG, Burton EC, McDonald KM, et al. Changes in rates of autopsy-detected diagnostic errors over time: a systematic review. JAMA 2003;289(21):2849–56.

7. Wittschieber D, Klauschen F, Kimmritz A-C, et al. Who is at risk for diagnostic discrepancies? Comparison of pre- and postmortal diagnoses in 1800 patients of 3 medical decades in East and West Berlin. PLoS One 2012;7(5):e37460.
8. Marshall HS, Milikowski C. Comparison of clinical diagnoses and autopsy findings: six-year retrospective study. Arch Pathol Lab Med 2017;141(9):1262–6.
9. Kuijpers CCHJ, Fronczek J, van de Goot FRW, et al. The value of autopsies in the era of high-tech medicine: discrepant findings persist. J Clin Pathol 2014;67(6):512–9.
10. Winters B, Custer J, Galvagno SMJ, et al. Diagnostic errors in the intensive care unit: a systematic review of autopsy studies. BMJ Qual Saf 2012;21(11):894–902.
11. Battle RM, Pathak D, Humble CG, et al. Factors influencing discrepancies between premortem and postmortem diagnoses. JAMA 1987;258(3):339–44.
12. Schwanda-Burger S, Moch H, Muntwyler J, et al. Diagnostic errors in the new millennium: a follow-up autopsy study. Mod Pathol 2012;25(6):777–83.
13. Fröhlich S, Ryan O, Murphy N, et al. Are autopsy findings still relevant to the management of critically ill patients in the modern era? Crit Care Med 2014;42(2):336–43.
14. Rusu S, Lavis P, Domingues Salgado V, et al. Comparison of antemortem clinical diagnosis and post-mortem findings in intensive care unit patients. Virchows Arch 2021;479(2):385–92.
15. Shojania KG, Burton EC. The vanishing nonforensic autopsy. N Engl J Med 2008; 358(9):873–5.
16. Maris C, Martin B, Creteur J, et al. Comparison of clinical and post-mortem findings in intensive care unit patients. Virchows Arch Int J Pathol 2007;450(3):329–33.
17. Dimopoulos G, Piagnerelli M, Berré J, et al. Post mortem examination in the intensive care unit: still useful? Intensive Care Med 2004;30(11):2080–5.
18. Liisanantti JH, Ala-Kokko TI. The impact of antemortem computed tomographic scanning on postmortem examination rate and frequency of missed diagnosis: a retrospective analysis of postmortem examination data. J Crit Care 2015; 30(6):1420.e1–4.
19. Tejerina EE, Padilla R, Abril E, et al. Autopsy-detected diagnostic errors over time in the intensive care unit. Hum Pathol 2018;76:85–90.
20. Custer JW, Winters BD, Goode V, et al. Diagnostic errors in the pediatric and neonatal ICU: a systematic review. Pediatr Crit Care Med 2015;16(1):29–36.
21. Cifra CL, Custer JW, Singh H, et al. Diagnostic errors in pediatric critical care: a systematic review. Pediatr Crit Care Med 2021;22(8):701–12.
22. Widmann R, Caduff R, Giudici L, et al. Value of postmortem studies in deceased neonatal and pediatric intensive care unit patients. Virchows Arch Int J Pathol 2017;470(2):217–23.
23. O'Rahelly M, McDermott M, Healy M. Autopsy and pre-mortem diagnostic discrepancy review in an Irish tertiary PICU. Eur J Pediatr 2021. https://doi.org/10.1007/s00431-021-04155-3.
24. Suzuki Y, Kume H, Togano T, et al. Epidemiology of visceral mycoses in autopsy cases in Japan: the data from 1989 to 2009 in the Annual of Pathological Autopsy Cases in Japan. Med Mycol 2013;51(5):522–6.
25. Lewis RE, Cahyame-Zuniga L, Leventakos K, et al. Epidemiology and sites of involvement of invasive fungal infections in patients with haematological malignancies: a 20-year autopsy study. Mycoses 2013;56(6):638–45.
26. Tejerina EE, Abril E, Padilla R, et al. Invasive aspergillosis in critically ill patients: an autopsy study. Mycoses 2019;62(8):673–9.
27. Blanco C, Steigman C, Probst N, et al. Discrepancies between autopsy and clinical findings among patients requiring extracorporeal membrane oxygenator support. ASAIO J 2014;60(2):207–10.

28. Multani A, Allard LS, Wangjam T, et al. Missed diagnosis and misdiagnosis of infectious diseases in hematopoietic cell transplant recipients: an autopsy study. Blood Adv 2019;3(22):3602–12.
29. Cagaanan AP, Aesif SW. Pulmonary complications after solid organ transplantation: an autopsy perspective. Transpl Proc 2018;50(10):3783–8.
30. Sharma S, Nadrous HF, Peters SG, et al. Pulmonary complications in adult blood and marrow transplant recipients: autopsy findings. Chest 2005;128(3):1385–92.
31. Khawaja O, Khalil M, Zmeili O, et al. Major discrepancies between clinical and postmortem diagnoses in critically ill cancer patients: is autopsy still useful? Avicenna J Med 2013;3(3):63–7.
32. Raghuram N, Alodan K, Bartels U, et al. Diagnostic discrepancies between antemortem clinical diagnosis and autopsy findings in pediatric cancer patients. Virchows Arch Int J Pathol 2021;478(6):1179–85.
33. Driessen RGH, Latten BGH, Bergmans DCJJ, et al. Clinical diagnoses vs. autopsy findings in early deceased septic patients in the intensive care: a retrospective cohort study. Virchows Arch Int J Pathol 2021;478(6):1173–8.
34. Fish J, Hartshorne N, Reay D, et al. The role of autopsy on patients with burns. J Burn Care Rehabil 2000;21(4):339–44.
35. Tsagkarakis M, Spyropoulou G-A, Pavlidis L, et al. Fatalities from a Greek Burn Unit-A clinicopathological correlation of 129 cases. Burns J Int Soc Burn Inj 2018;44(1):226–9.
36. Tejerina E, Esteban A, Fernández-Segoviano P, et al. Accuracy of clinical definitions of ventilator-associated pneumonia: comparison with autopsy findings. J Crit Care 2010;25(1):62–8.
37. Leape LL, Brennan TA, Laird N, et al. The nature of adverse events in hospitalized patients. Results of the Harvard Medical Practice Study II. N Engl J Med 1991;324(6):377–84.
38. McGloin H, Adam SK, Singer M. Unexpected deaths and referrals to intensive care of patients on general wards. Are some cases potentially avoidable? J R Coll Physicians Lond 1999;33(3):255–9.
39. Lehmann LS, Puopolo AL, Shaykevich S, et al. Iatrogenic events resulting in intensive care admission: frequency, cause, and disclosure to patients and institutions. Am J Med 2005;118(4):409–13.
40. Marquet K, Claes N, De Troy E, et al. One fourth of unplanned transfers to a higher level of care are associated with a highly preventable adverse event: a patient record review in six Belgian hospitals. Crit Care Med 2015;43(5):1053–61.
41. Davalos MC, Samuels K, Meyer AND, et al. Finding diagnostic errors in children admitted to the PICU. Pediatr Crit Care Med 2017;18(3):265–71.
42. Bergl PA, Taneja A, El-Kareh R, et al. Frequency, risk factors, causes, and consequences of diagnostic errors in critically ill medical patients: a retrospective cohort study. Crit Care Med 2019;47(11):e902–10.
43. Cifra CL, Ten Eyck P, Dawson JD, et al. Factors associated with diagnostic error on admission to a PICU: a pilot study. Pediatr Crit Care Med 2020;21(5):e311–5.
44. Singh H, Sittig DF. Advancing the science of measurement of diagnostic errors in healthcare: the Safer Dx framework. BMJ Qual Saf 2015;24(2):103–10.
45. Singh H, Khanna A, Spitzmueller C, et al. Recommendations for using the revised safer Dx Instrument to help measure and improve diagnostic safety. Diagn Berl Ger 2019;6(4):315–23.
46. Al-Mutairi A, Meyer AND, Thomas EJ, et al. Accuracy of the safer Dx instrument to identify diagnostic errors in primary care. J Gen Intern Med 2016;31(6):602–8.

47. Gunderson CG, Bilan VP, Holleck JL, et al. Prevalence of harmful diagnostic errors in hospitalised adults: a systematic review and meta-analysis. BMJ Qual Saf 2020;29(12):1008–18.
48. Newman-Toker DE, Wang Z, Zhu Y, et al. Rate of diagnostic errors and serious misdiagnosis-related harms for major vascular events, infections, and cancers: toward a national incidence estimate using the "Big Three". Diagn Berl Ger 2021;8(1):67–84.
49. Newman-Toker DE, Schaffer AC, Yu-Moe CW, et al. Serious misdiagnosis-related harms in malpractice claims: the "Big Three" - vascular events, infections, and cancers. Diagn Berl Ger 2019;6(3):227–40.
50. Sauter TC, Capaldo G, Hoffmann M, et al. Non-specific complaints at emergency department presentation result in unclear diagnoses and lengthened hospitalization: a prospective observational study. Scand J Trauma Resusc Emerg Med 2018;26(1):60.
51. Hautz WE, Kämmer JE, Hautz SC, et al. Diagnostic error increases mortality and length of hospital stay in patients presenting through the emergency room. Scand J Trauma Resusc Emerg Med 2019;27(1):54.
52. Saber Tehrani AS, Lee H, Mathews SC, et al. 25-year summary of US malpractice claims for diagnostic errors 1986-2010: an analysis from the National Practitioner Data Bank. BMJ Qual Saf 2013;22(8):672–80.
53. Durning SJ, Artino AR. Situativity theory: a perspective on how participants and the environment can interact: AMEE Guide no. 52. Med Teach 2011;33(3):188–99.
54. Konopasky A, Artino AR, Battista A, et al. Understanding context specificity: the effect of contextual factors on clinical reasoning. Diagn Berl Ger 2020;7(3):257–64.
55. Weiner SJ, Schwartz A, Weaver F, et al. Contextual errors and failures in individualizing patient care: a multicenter study. Ann Intern Med 2010;153(2):69–75.
56. Rhee C, Kadri SS, Danner RL, et al. Diagnosing sepsis is subjective and highly variable: a survey of intensivists using case vignettes. Crit Care Lond Engl 2016;20:89.
57. Filbin MR, Lynch J, Gillingham TD, et al. Presenting symptoms independently Predict mortality in septic shock: Importance of a previously Unmeasured confounder. Crit Care Med 2018;46(10):1592–9.
58. Aaronson E, Jansson P, Wittbold K, et al. Unscheduled return visits to the emergency department with ICU admission: a trigger tool for diagnostic error. Am J Emerg Med 2020;38(8):1584–7.
59. Raffel KE, Kantor MA, Barish P, et al. Prevalence and characterisation of diagnostic error among 7-day all-cause hospital medicine readmissions: a retrospective cohort study. BMJ Qual Saf 2020;29(12):971–9.
60. Podbregar M, Voga G, Krivec B, et al. Should we confirm our clinical diagnostic certainty by autopsies? Intensive Care Med 2001;27(11):1750–5.
61. ALQahtani DA, Rotgans JI, Mamede S, et al. Factors underlying suboptimal diagnostic performance in physicians under time pressure. Med Educ 2018;52(12):1288–98.
62. Chopra V, Harrod M, Winter S, et al. Focused ethnography of diagnosis in academic medical centers. J Hosp Med 2018;13(10):668–72.
63. Wagner J, Gabler NB, Ratcliffe SJ, et al. Outcomes among patients discharged from busy intensive care units. Ann Intern Med 2013;159(7):447–55.
64. Eriksson CO, Stoner RC, Eden KB, et al. The association between hospital capacity strain and inpatient outcomes in highly developed countries: a systematic review. J Gen Intern Med 2017;32(6):686–96.

Dual Process Theory and Cognitive Load

How Intensivists Make Diagnoses

Emily Harris, MD, Lekshmi Santhosh, MD, MAEd*

KEYWORDS

- Diagnostic reasoning ● Clinical reasoning ● ICU ● Dual process theory
- Cognitive load

KEY POINTS

- Clinical reasoning in the intensive care unit (ICU) can be modeled by dual process theory, among other theories.
- Physicians in the ICU often switch between system 1 and system 2 processing and use both systems simultaneously.
- Cognitive load affects how easily and readily physicians switch between system 1 and system 2 processing.

INTRODUCTION

More than 20 years ago, the Institute of Medicine highlighted the remarkable prevalence of medical errors with the landmark *To Err Is Human* report.[1] Diagnostic errors have been defined as the failure to establish an accurate or timely explanation for the patient's health problems or effectively communicate the explanation to the patient; the estimated frequency of such errors in high acuity settings is at least 5% to 10%. A retrospective study of patients admitted to National Health Service hospitals found that 5.1% of medical errors were due to diagnostic errors.[2] Another study of intensive care unit (ICU) admissions found that diagnostic errors were present in 7% of ICU admissions. All these errors caused patient harm, and only 33% were recognized by the ICU team within 24 hours of occurrence.[3] Because of the prevalence of diagnostic errors and their associated harm, there has been great interest in reducing errors by improving clinicians' diagnostic reasoning.

There are many clinical reasoning frameworks that may apply to the fast-paced ICU clinical learning environment. For example, clinical reasoning in the ICU can be

University of California San Francisco, 505 Parnassus Avenue, Box 0111, San Francisco, CA 94117, USA
* Corresponding author.
E-mail address: lekshmi.santhosh@ucsf.edu

Crit Care Clin 38 (2022) 27–36
https://doi.org/10.1016/j.ccc.2021.07.001
0749-0704/22/© 2021 Elsevier Inc. All rights reserved.

criticalcare.theclinics.com

modeled by dual process reasoning, in which a clinician toggles between intuition and deliberate analysis depending on patient, environmental, and individual factors. Cognitive load also plays a pivotal role in providing care in the ICU, and strategies to reduce cognitive load can allow physicians to optimize their clinical reasoning. In addition, techniques, such as deliberate diagnostic pauses and reflection, can allow physicians to facilitate switching from system 1 to system 2 processing when appropriate and may help improve diagnostic reasoning in the high-pressure environment of the ICU. In this article, the authors highlight these frameworks and their applicability to the ICU clinical learning environment.

MODELS OF DIAGNOSTIC REASONING

Several groups proposed models of cognition and reasoning comprising 2 processing systems beginning in the 1970s, including Wason and Evans as well as Tversky and Kahneman.[4,5] These models, which were developed in parallel, have come to be known as dual process theory.[6] The core tenet of dual process theory is the existence of 2 distinct systems of reasoning. The first, system 1, is often referred to as "intuitive" or "automatic." It uses pattern recognition and association to arrive at a conclusion quickly. System 2 processing is often referred to as "analytical." It relies more heavily on rules, deduction, and active reasoning. Subsequent behavioral studies have supported dual process theory in matching and discrimination tasks.[7] Studies using functional MRI have shown activation of different neural pathways when speed versus accuracy are emphasized during behavioral tasks.[8]

Since its initial description, dual process theory has become an important model for clinical reasoning.[9,10] Depending on the situation, individuals may use system 1 or system 2 processing. In the realm of clinical reasoning, system 1 processing frequently uses mental shortcuts, such as illness scripts or heuristics. For example, a physician encountering a patient with chest pain, an elevated troponin, and ST segment elevation on electrocardiogram would quickly diagnose a myocardial infarction via system 1 processing. System 2 processing is thought to be used in clinical situations in which no clear pattern has emerged or is recognized. For example, a physician encountering a patient with generalized abdominal pain will undertake a more systematic and thorough diagnostic evaluation. This evaluation will take more time and require more cognitive expenditure.

Neither system 1 nor system 2 processing is thought to be superior in its diagnostic accuracy.[6,11] However, one may have benefit over the other depending on the situation. For example, a physician encountering an easily recognizable clinical syndrome presenting in a classic way (for example, the aforementioned patient with myocardial infarction) may rely more on system 1 processing to diagnose the patient. In this type of situation with an easily recognizable pattern, the physician could conserve cognitive energy in making a diagnosis. The resource-intensive process of undergoing an extensive workup is also avoided, as the appropriate testing can quickly be identified. Using system 1 processing in this situation often is quite accurate: for example, Barrows and colleagues[12] found that when physicians generated a correct diagnosis in the first 5 minutes of a clinical encounter, eventual accuracy was 98%. On the other hand, a physician encountering the patient with generalized abdominal pain will likely rely more on system 2 processing. This presentation could be a manifestation of many pathologic processes, and the physician is unable to quickly recognize a characteristic pattern associated with a particular disease. This uncertainty may nudge the physician to use more systematic reasoning, consider the patient's history and data more thoroughly, and order appropriate additional diagnostic studies.

In Croskerry's model[9] of dual process theory, he proposes a "toggle function," which allows physicians to switch between system 1 and system 2 reasoning when needed. Toggling from intuition to analytical thinking may be warranted when clinical situations evolve and require further reflection and reasoning, such as when the patient does not respond to treatment of the presumptive diagnosis. Similarly, a complex case can often be distilled into a more simplified problem, such as acute hypoxemic respiratory failure or distributive shock, which can then activate more intuitive reasoning. In essence, clinicians tend toward system 1 reasoning in situations with recognizable patterns and system 2 reasoning in situations where no clear pattern is recognized but fluidly transition between both systems depending on a large number of cognitive, environmental, and other task-related factors.

COGNITIVE LOAD THEORY

Cognitive load theory describes how individuals use different parts of their memory. Three types of memory exist according to cognitive load theory: sensory memory, long-term memory, and working memory.[13] Sensory memory and long-term memory hold information in the long term for later recall. Working memory is used to manipulate stored information and new information and is essential in learning. Although sensory memory and long-term memory have an infinite capacity to store information, working memory does not. Working memory can hold a limited amount of information at a time; when the strain on working memory exceeds capacity, people may not be able to store new information in long-term memory.

Because the capacity of working memory is finite, it is susceptible to strain when it holds too many pieces of information at once.[14] The amount of information occupying working memory at any 1 time is referred to as cognitive load. Three categories of load can place strain on working memory capacity: intrinsic load, extrinsic load, and germane load.[15] Intrinsic load is composed of cognitive demands that are essential to the task at hand. For example, when inserting a central venous catheter, the clinician must observe sterile technique and ensure that no contamination takes place; these aspects of the procedure put strain on working memory. Extrinsic load is information that is not essential to the task at hand. A colleague asking a question about an unrelated matter while the clinician is inserting a central venous catheter is an example of extrinsic load. Last, germane load refers to information that will be stored as part of a framework for future long-term memory; for example, a learner spends time manipulating the ultrasound probe to visualize the internal jugular vein and carotid artery before insertion to familiarize themselves with the orientation.

A variety of factors unique to the ICU place strain on the working memory capacity of clinicians. High patient acuity requiring many management decisions increases intrinsic load in the ICU. More subtle factors, like electronic medical records, communicating plans for patient care with colleagues, and donning and doffing of personal protective equipment, also place a strain on intrinsic cognitive load.[16,17] There is also a high burden of distraction in the ICU; 1 study found 4.36 distractions per doctor per hour in the ICU. Many of these distractions were from other physicians (35%) and nurses (30%).[18] These distractions place extraneous strain on cognitive load. For trainees who may be unfamiliar with the ICU environment, systems, or patient acuity, all of these factors also come with increased germane load as they navigate new terrain.

When the strain placed by cognitive load exceeds the capacity of working memory, clinicians experience cognitive overload.[19] Cognitive overload interferes with executive processing tasks and learning in behavioral studies.[15,20] It may interfere with interpersonal interactions and procedural skill learning as well.[21,22]

DIAGNOSTIC UNCERTAINTY IN THE INTENSIVE CARE UNIT

Environmental and systems factors in the ICU affect cognitive load and clinicians' ability to manipulate new information in their working memory. However, they are not the only factors to affect clinical reasoning in the ICU. Other affective factors, including physician mood, fatigue, confidence, and experience, all play a role in clinical reasoning. A second-year resident working a 24-hour shift is likely to experience fatigue, stress, and lower confidence than a seasoned attending. In the hospital setting, diagnostic uncertainty is common, and in 1 study, 30% of physicians ordered additional diagnostic tests "to be safe."[23] In the ICU, patients have higher medical acuity, and physicians are frequently tasked with caring for patients with undifferentiated illnesses. In this situation, diagnostic certainty may be even lower.

One model of diagnostic certainty proposed 3 major categories of uncertainty.[24] Technical uncertainty involves having inadequate data, for example, not knowing the sensitivity of a test to detect a diagnosis. Personal uncertainty encompasses uncertainty regarding a patient's wishes, such as not knowing whether a patient would want life-sustaining treatment like mechanical ventilation. Conceptual uncertainty involves the difficult nature of applying abstract concepts like diagnostic criteria to a real-life patient presentation, for example, diagnosing adult-onset Still disease in a patient with high fever, headache, altered mental status, and lymphadenopathy. Because of the nature of medical problems, these diagnostic uncertainties are all common. Furthermore, diagnostic accuracy, whether a diagnosis is correct, is distinct from diagnostic certainty, and the two may not be aligned in a clinician's mind. In 1 autopsy study, 17% of patients who died in an ICU were found to have incorrect diagnoses on autopsy.[25]

It may be helpful to consider a 2 × 2 model whereby diagnostic certainty and diagnostic accuracy are considered separately[26] (**Fig. 1**). This model may be used to conceptualize and communicate a clinician's sense of diagnostic certainty and accuracy to other members of a care team. For example, in a straightforward case of sepsis from a urinary source, they might identify that they are within quadrant 1, that is, certain and accurate. On the other hand, a less straightforward case of unexplained altered mental status may fall into quadrant 3 (uncertain and inaccurate).

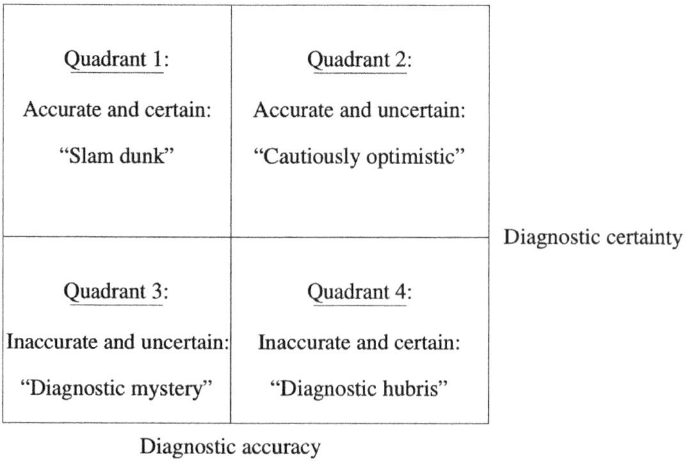

Quadrant 1: Accurate and certain: "Slam dunk"	Quadrant 2: Accurate and uncertain: "Cautiously optimistic"	
Quadrant 3: Inaccurate and uncertain: "Diagnostic mystery"	Quadrant 4: Inaccurate and certain: "Diagnostic hubris"	Diagnostic certainty

Diagnostic accuracy

Fig. 1. Proposed model considering diagnostic accuracy versus certainty.

System 1 processing is an advantageous approach to diagnostic reasoning in situations in which certainty and accuracy are both high (quadrant 1). In these scenarios, physicians diagnose patients by recognizing distinct patterns already stored in their long-term memory, and accessing this memory requires minimal cognitive load. As a result, physicians retain greater capacity in their working memory for other complex reasoning and tasks. By contrast, using system 2 processing in these situations may unnecessarily increase cognitive load burden, lengthen time to diagnosis, and could lead to additional and costly testing.

When either diagnostic certainty or accuracy is low, using system 1 has the potential to lead to missed or wrong diagnosis. In these situations, data commonly do not fit cleanly within the criteria or pattern for any 1 disease, or the applicability of existing data may be uncertain. System 2 processing may prove more advantageous in these scenarios. Rather than attempting to fit existing data into a preexisting schema (which may lead to ignoring conflicting evidence), system 2 processing allows reconsideration of available information. Narrative data suggest that physicians use system 1 processing, also known as clinical intuition, to recognize when available information does not fit with the presumed diagnosis.[27] As mentioned, this recognition may prompt the physician to toggle to system 2 processing, which allows review of data and initiates a broader diagnostic workup.[9]

FINDING BALANCE

In an ideal world, physicians would use system 1 and system 2 processing appropriately in order to minimize cognitive overload and maximize diagnostic accuracy and certainty. However, medical problems are not clearly defined, and physicians discover information and details over time.[28] Because of the imprecise nature of medical presentations and the fact that cases unfold over time, it is often favorable to switch between systems of processing as additional information becomes available. For example, a patient may present with fever and circulatory shock requiring vasopressors. Initially, the physician uses system 1 processing to manage resuscitation and initiate vasopressors, presuming that this presentation is likely septic shock. However, when the clinician fails to find a potential infectious source, yet a high vasopressor requirement persists, the physician will likely switch to system 2 thinking and will systematically consider other causes of shock, including cardiogenic, anaphylactic, neurogenic, and obstructive. They may also obtain additional diagnostic information. By switching to system 2 thinking when the data do not agree with the initial diagnosis, the physician can enhance diagnostic certainty and accuracy.

Because of the high acuity and high stakes involved in caring for critically ill patients, physicians in the ICU often conduct diagnosis and management simultaneously. This style of practice forces the use of system 1 and system 2 processing in parallel or in very quick succession. For example, in the patient with fever and shock, the physician will likely give fluids and start antibiotics using system 1 processing, which recognizes the likely syndrome of sepsis. However, because of the risk of missing one of the other potential causes of shock, the physician will quickly (or even simultaneously) use system 2 processing to evaluate for other causes. The risk of morbidity and mortality to the patient is very high if the physician waits 48 hours until negative cultures return before rapidly and serially ruling out other causes of shock; thus, there is a tendency toward rapid intuitive management of sepsis. However, the clinician often will use system 2 processing concurrently with giving fluids and antibiotics by using ultrasound to evaluate for signs of depressed cardiac function or volume overload, suggesting cardiogenic shock or a pericardial effusion, suggesting obstructive shock.

Subsequent findings of a small and collapsible inferior vena cava on ultrasound and high central venous oxygen saturation could increase the certainty of the initial working diagnosis of septic shock, which is technically a deliberative system 2 task that supports system 1's intuition.

In other situations, clinicians may not switch from system 1 to system 2 thinking despite the fact that it would be advantageous. Why do clinicians fail to switch from system 1 to system 2, even when there is information suggesting that their initial gestalt or intuition was incorrect?

One reason behind failure to switch to a more analytical form of reasoning may be cognitive overload. Cognitively overloaded physicians may be unable to recognize new information that contradicts their current diagnosis. One review found that cognitive load was inversely associated with performance.[19] It also interferes with other executive functions on behavioral tasks.[20] There may be a situation in which a physician initially used system 1 processing to diagnose a patient. However, new data and information arose later on in the patient's course, whether hours or days. Now, the physician is cognitively overloaded and is unable to recognize that this new information contradicts their original diagnosis. If they had recognized that, they might have switched to system 2 processing to approach the patient in a more systematic and analytical way to arrive at a more accurate diagnosis with greater certainty. Indeed, interviews with attending physicians suggest that trainees who are cognitively overloaded are less likely to synthesize information appropriately and may give inaccurate assessments of patients.[21]

Another cause of failure to switch from system 1 to system 2 processing when appropriate is lack of experience or expertise. Although evidence suggests that expertise is protective from cognitive overload, expertise also appears to allow physicians to more accurately evaluate their own diagnostic certainty and accuracy.[19] In a study involving hypothetical case scenarios, resident physicians were overconfident in their diagnosis more frequently than attending physicians.[29] This state of overconfidence can be represented by quadrant 4 in the 2×2 table: "diagnostic hubris," in which a clinician is inaccurate but certain of their diagnosis. In this situation, physicians are unlikely to recognize inaccuracy or switch from system 1 to system 2 thinking when it is appropriate. With experience and feedback on diagnostic outcomes, clinicians may be better able to align their diagnostic confidence and accuracy or improve their diagnostic calibration.[30]

STRATEGIES FOR SWITCHING BETWEEN SYSTEMS

Given the importance of using the 2 systems of processing at appropriate times in order to maximize accuracy and minimize cognitive load, how can clinicians strategically use each system when most appropriate?

Reducing cognitive load to increase working memory availability is 1 way to facilitate recognition of incongruous or new information that may affect diagnosis and to allow physicians to recognize when switching to system 2 processing would be advantageous. One relatively simple solution is to optimize the work environment to avoid extraneous cognitive strain; examples might include avoiding interruptions during procedures or team discussions with nonemergent questions. Smaller changes, such as displaying information in easier-to-interpret formats in the medical record, has also been shown to reduce cognitive load.[16] Similarly, the very act of writing out key diagnostic data points on a whiteboard to see how data points might connect is another way to explicitly manage a clinician's cognitive load and also to distribute this cognitive load to the team effectively.

Other strategies for optimizing the electronic medical record to reduce cognitive load might include ready-made order sets, which include orders for standard tasks. For example, in intubated patients, the order set may include an order for a daily spontaneous breathing trial (SBT). This automation removes the cognitive load of remembering to order an SBT from the physician. Delegating tasks to other professionals on the care team may also decrease cognitive load. For example, pharmacists may be able to help with deep vein thrombosis prophylaxis dosing or monitoring vancomycin levels. Diagnostically, development of schemas for common problems, such as standard approaches to new hypoxemic respiratory failure, hypotension/shock, and thrombocytopenia, may allow clinicians to quickly review data and tests without cognitive overload.

Another strategy for facilitating switching from system 1 to system 2 is the diagnostic pause or timeout. Inspired by preprocedural timeouts, a diagnostic pause has been described as "reflect on the current working diagnosis and the evidence supporting that diagnosis."[31] Beyond reflection and review of information, checklists have also been proposed as a format for diagnostic pauses.[32,33] Regardless of the mechanism, a diagnostic pause integrates a mechanism for forcing physicians to switch to type 2 thinking by examining all information and data available. It is also an opportunity to identify any uncertainty in diagnosis and ultimately change course if warranted. A study of diagnostic pauses in the ambulatory setting found that diagnostic pauses led to additional or different tests being ordered for 13% of patients.[34] Some investigators have also argued that the ICU-to-ward transition is a particularly high-risk time and that the deliberate inclusion of a diagnostic pause in this transition period would be beneficial in reducing diagnostic errors or delays (Lekshmi Santhosh, unpublished data, 2021).

Last, studies have also shown that physicians who are more self-reflective may have better patient outcomes.[35] The cause behind this is unclear. However, it may be that physicians who are more reflective are conducting frequent, internal diagnostic pauses. Their reflective nature allows them to frequently audit which processing system they are using and to switch from system 1 to system 2 when appropriate. It also appears that interventions aimed at instructing self-reflection and promoting reflection for physicians can improve diagnostic reasoning.[36,37] Similarly, this improvement may encourage physicians who are more reflective to conduct cognitive autopsies. During a cognitive autopsy, a physician might reflect on aspects of a case that went well, what went poorly, and whether there are any clinical pearls or learning that might improve diagnostic processes in future practice.[38] This procedure can also be thought of as reflecting on ways to reduce the germane load in future cases. For example, in a case of late diagnosis of cardiogenic shock, which was mistaken for septic shock, the physician might reflect on the fact that the recognition of shock and early supportive measures were effective, but that their initial volume examination was not accurate and that the addition of point-of-care ultrasound earlier in the hospital course may improve their diagnostic efficacy in the future.

SUMMARY

Diagnostic errors have been shown to occur frequently across health care settings, including the ICU. Factors contributing to diagnostic errors include physician, patient, and environmental factors. Central to all of these is the diagnostic reasoning process, which is most frequently modeled by dual process theory. Although neither system 1 nor system 2 is clearly superior in improving diagnostic accuracy, each system carries advantages in certain circumstances. Furthermore, there are many situations in which it is advantageous to switch from system 1 to system 2. In the ICU setting, using system 1 and system 2 processing simultaneously or in quick succession is often necessary. Use of system 1 versus system 2 thinking depends on a variety of factors but may be influenced by cognitive load and expertise of the clinician. Strategies and tools such as diagnostic pauses or timeouts and self-reflection may facilitate switching between system 1 and system 2 thinking when necessary, allowing physicians to reduce diagnostic error rates. Furthermore, clinicians can build long-term diagnostic reasoning skills that allow them to more effectively manage their cognitive load.

CLINICS CARE POINTS

- Consider how physician, patient, and environmental factors might contribute to diagnostic errors in the intensive care unit.
- Neither system 1 nor system 2 thinking are superior in improving diagnostic accuracy; consider reflecting on the advantages of each system in different circumstances.
- Use tools such as diagnostic pauses or timeouts and self-reflection to facilitate switching between system 1 and system 2 thinking.

DISCLOSURE

Neither author has any commercial or financial conflict of interest to disclose.

REFERENCES

1. Donaldson MS, Corrigan JM, Kohn LT. To err is human: building a safer health system. 2000.
2. Sari AB, Sheldon TA, Cracknell A, et al. Extent, nature and consequences of adverse events: results of a retrospective casenote review in a large NHS hospital. Qual Saf Health Care 2007;16(6):434–9.
3. Bergl PA, Taneja A, El-Kareh R, et al. Frequency, risk factors, causes, and consequences of diagnostic errors in critically ill medical patients: a retrospective cohort study. Crit Care Med 2019;47(11):e902–10.
4. Wason PC, Evans BT. Dual processes in reasoning? Cognition 1974;3(2):141–54.
5. Tversky A, Kahneman D. Judgment under uncertainty: heuristics and biases. Science 1974;185(4157):1124–31.
6. Evans JS. Dual-processing accounts of reasoning, judgment, and social cognition. Annu Rev Psychol 2008;59:255–78.
7. Yin Y, Yu T, Wang S, et al. Event-related potentials support a dual process account of the Embedded Chinese Character Task. Neuropsychologia 2018;121: 186–92.
8. Ivanoff J, Branning P, Marois R. fMRI evidence for a dual process account of the speed-accuracy tradeoff in decision-making. PLoS One 2008;3(7):e2635.
9. Croskerry P. A universal model of diagnostic reasoning. Acad Med 2009;84(8): 1022–8.
10. Marcum JA. An integrated model of clinical reasoning: dual-process theory of cognition and metacognition. J Eval Clin Pract 2012;18(5):954–61.
11. Norman G. Dual processing and diagnostic errors. Adv Health Sci Educ Theor Pract 2009;14(Suppl 1):37–49.
12. Barrows HS, Norman GR, Neufeld VR, et al. The clinical reasoning of randomly selected physicians in general medical practice. Clin Invest Med 1982;5(1): 49–55.

13. Mancinetti M, Guttormsen S, Berendonk C. Cognitive load in internal medicine: what every clinical teacher should know about cognitive load theory. Eur J Intern Med 2019;60:4–8.
14. Baddeley A. Working memory: theories, models, and controversies. Annu Rev Psychol 2012;63:1–29.
15. Young JQ, Van Merrienboer J, Durning S, et al. Cognitive load theory: implications for medical education: AMEE guide no. 86. Med Teach 2014;36(5):371–84.
16. Ahmed A, Chandra S, Herasevich V, et al. The effect of two different electronic health record user interfaces on intensive care provider task load, errors of cognition, and performance. Crit Care Med 2011;39(7):1626–34.
17. Díaz-Guio DA, Ricardo-Zapata A, Ospina-Velez J, et al. Cognitive load and performance of health care professionals in donning and doffing PPE before and after a simulation-based educational intervention and its implications during the COVID-19 pandemic for biosafety. Infez Med 2020;28(suppl 1):111–7.
18. See KC, Phua J, Mukhopadhyay A, et al. Characteristics of distractions in the intensive care unit: how serious are they and who are at risk? Singapore Med J 2014;55(7):358–62.
19. Sewell JL, Maggio LA, Ten Cate O, et al. Cognitive load theory for training health professionals in the workplace: a BEME review of studies among diverse professions: BEME guide no. 53. Med Teach 2019;41(3):256–70.
20. Schneider D, Lam R, Bayliss AP, et al. Cognitive load disrupts implicit theory-of-mind processing. Psychol Sci 2012;23(8):842–7.
21. Sewell JL, Santhosh L, O'Sullivan PS. How do attending physicians describe cognitive overload among their workplace learners? Med Educ 2020;54(12):1129–36.
22. Sewell JL, Boscardin CK, Young JQ, et al. Learner, patient, and supervisor features are associated with different types of cognitive load during procedural skills training: implications for teaching and instructional design. Acad Med 2017;92(11):1622–31.
23. Wray CM, Cho HJ. Web exclusive. Annals for hospitalists inpatient notes - medical uncertainty as a driver of resource use-examining the "gray zones" of clinical care. Ann Intern Med 2018;168(12):HO2–3.
24. Beresford EB. Uncertainty and the shaping of medical decisions. Hastings Cent Rep 1991;21(4):6–11.
25. Tejerina EE, Padilla R, Abril E, et al. Autopsy-detected diagnostic errors over time in the intensive care unit. Hum Pathol 2018;76:85–90.
26. Santhosh L, Chou CL, Connor DM. Diagnostic uncertainty: from education to communication. Diagnosis 2019;6(2):121–6.
27. Vanstone M, Monteiro S, Colvin E, et al. Experienced physician descriptions of intuition in clinical reasoning: a typology. Diagnosis (Berl) 2019;6(3):259–68.
28. Barrows HS, Feltovich PJ. The clinical reasoning process. Med Educ 1987;21(2):86–91.
29. Friedman CP, Gatti GG, Franz TM, et al. Do physicians know when their diagnoses are correct? Implications for decision support and error reduction. J Gen Intern Med 2005;20(4):334–9.
30. Meyer AND, Singh H. The path to diagnostic excellence includes feedback to calibrate how clinicians think. JAMA 2019;321(8):737–8.
31. Trowbridge RL. Twelve tips for teaching avoidance of diagnostic errors. Med Teach 2008;30(5):496–500.
32. Ely JW, Graber ML, Croskerry P. Checklists to reduce diagnostic errors. Acad Med 2011;86(3):307–13.

33. Winters BD, Aswani MS, Pronovost PJ. Commentary: reducing diagnostic errors: another role for checklists? Acad Med 2011;86(3):279–81.
34. Huang GC, Kriegel G, Wheaton C, et al. Implementation of diagnostic pauses in the ambulatory setting. BMJ Qual Saf 2018;27(6):492–7.
35. Novack DH, Suchman AL, Clark W, et al. Calibrating the physician. Personal awareness and effective patient care. Working group on promoting physician personal awareness, American Academy on Physician and Patient. JAMA 1997;278(6):502–9.
36. Lambe KA, O'Reilly G, Kelly BD, et al. Dual-process cognitive interventions to enhance diagnostic reasoning: a systematic review. BMJ Qual Saf 2016;25(10): 808–20.
37. Mamede S, Hautz WE, Berendonk C, et al. Think twice: effects on diagnostic accuracy of returning to the case to reflect upon the initial diagnosis. Acad Med 2020;95(8):1223–9.
38. Mehdi A, Foshee C, Green W, et al. Cognitive autopsy: a transformative group approach to mitigate cognitive bias. J Grad Med Educ 2018;10(3):345–7.

Decision Making
Healthy Heuristics and Betraying Biases

Courtney W. Mangus, MD*, Prashant Mahajan, MD, MPH, MBA

KEYWORDS

- Heuristics • Cognition • Bias • Cognitive dispositions to respond • Diagnostic error

KEY POINTS

- Heuristics are mental shortcuts that allow for decisions to be made efficiently and accurately under stress, time-constraints, high cognitive load, and large decision density.
- Heuristics often lead to accurate conclusions and correct diagnoses, but can be prone to failure.
- Failed heuristics are described as cognitive biases or cognitive dispositions to respond.
- Many cognitive biases relevant to the practice of medicine have been described, and ongoing research seeks to better understand their role in diagnosis and devise strategies to prevent cognitive error.

INTRODUCTION

An experienced clinician enters a young patient's room and, within moments, usually has a good sense as to how ill the patient may be. The child who is alert, bright-eyed, active, and eating animal crackers is almost certainly not sick. The toddler who is quiet, pale, listless, and unaffected when a stranger approaches is likely ill or injured and in need of medical attention. These conclusions drawn from a first impression, or *gestalt*, inform many subsequent decisions. Of course, the clinician will perform a history and physical examination, but their gestalt will influence their decision making. Here, the authors explore how gestalt, intuitive reasoning, and decisional shortcuts (*heuristics*) influence medical decision making and clinical diagnosis, especially in the emergency and critical care settings. The authors describe the role of cognitive biases in diagnostic error and conclude with a summary of strategies to mitigate bias and future research directions to enhance diagnostic safety.

Departments of Emergency Medicine and Pediatrics, University of Michigan, 1540 East Hospital Drive, CW 2-737, SPC 4260, Ann Arbor, MI 48109-4260, USA
* Corresponding author.
E-mail address: cmangus@med.umich.edu

Crit Care Clin 38 (2022) 37–49
https://doi.org/10.1016/j.ccc.2021.07.002
criticalcare.theclinics.com
0749-0704/22/© 2021 Elsevier Inc. All rights reserved.

BACKGROUND: HOW DECISIONS ARE MADE

Dual process theory is the preeminent model used to explain human reasoning and decision making.[1,2] It describes two interrelated cognitive systems at play when the human brain makes a decision (**Table 1**). System 1 is intuitive: it is the brain's automatic, knee-jerk response to a problem it has encountered before. It is based on pattern recognition and previous experiences. Consider a simple example: when asked the sum of 2 + 2, the mature human brain responds with the correct answer without thinking or performing a mental calculation. The answer is there subconsciously and provided involuntarily.[1–3]

In contrast, system 2 is analytical and deliberate. When the brain confronts a complex decision or a problem it has not previously encountered, it intentionally slows down to methodically analyze and process the issue at hand. This process requires dedicated, critical thinking and more time than the system 1 approach. It is applied to complicated problems or those whereby there is no prior experience to guide decision making, such as when a novice clinician encounters a common but personally unfamiliar clinical presentation.[1,3]

The two systems do not operate entirely independently or without overlap. It has been proposed that they operate within a "cognitive continuum" wherein the mind oscillates between system 1 and system 2 type of thinking, resulting in variable efficiency and accuracy in decision making.[1,4]

SYSTEM 1 THINKING AND MEDICAL DECISION MAKING

In the last few decades, dual process theory has been applied to medical decision making and clinical diagnosis. In the clinical setting, system 1 thinking is used more frequently than its deliberative counterpart.[5,6] Here, the clinician recognizes the salient features of a patient's presentation and can make a diagnosis or clinical decision intuitively and expeditiously. This type of reasoning is efficient and usually accurate when the patient's presentation follows a known disease script, and its features are pathognomonic.[1] Notably, as clinicians gain experience, their repertoire of presentations and disease scripts increases. Consequently, there are a growing number of clinical scenarios whereby heuristics may be used, and seasoned clinicians increasingly use more intuitive decision making while reducing their cognitive load.

Intuitive decision making is invaluable in dynamic settings, such as the emergency department (ED) and intensive care unit (ICU), where lack of time, multiple competing priorities, and heavy cognitive load are an inherent part of this complex clinical environment. Several aspects of clinical care in this setting present unique challenges to accurate and timely diagnosis. Clinicians often operate with limited prior knowledge of the patient and their medical history, and many critically ill patients present altered,

Table 1	
Characteristics of system 1 and system 2 thinking	
System 1 = Intuitive	**System 2 = Analytical**
Automatic, subconscious, involuntary	Slow, methodical, deliberate
Relies on patterns and previous experience	Requires critical thinking
Cognitive ease	Cognitive strain
Susceptible to error and bias	Less susceptible to bias
Rapid	Time-consuming

obtunded, or otherwise unable to participate in their own care. In addition, clinicians practicing in critical care settings are prone to stress, distractions, sleep deprivation, and burnout—suboptimal conditions that predispose to intuitive thinking rather than analytical decision making.[1,7] These same conditions and use of system 1 thinking may also predispose to bias and diagnostic error, which will be reviewed in greater detail in later discussion.

Despite potential flaws, intuitive decision making often prevails in settings like the ICU or ED. It is this type of decision making that allows a clinician to encounter a patient in extremis and act intuitively and instantly to provide life-saving care. With just a cursory assessment of the patient and perhaps a glance at the cardiac monitor, a proficient clinician in a critical care setting will instinctually implement fluid resuscitation, respiratory support, defibrillation, or pharmacologic interventions (eg, antiarrhythmics, antiepileptics, antibiotics) and stabilize the patient. In these critical moments, there is little time for methodical analysis, and intuitive reasoning often prevails. Deliberate thought and careful contemplation are rarely required and, in some instances, may be detrimental if they delay implementation of life-saving interventions.

HEURISTICS AND BIAS

At the heart of system 1 thinking are *heuristics*. Heuristics are mental shortcuts based on intuitive thinking, pattern recognition, and prior experience. The study of heuristics, decision making, and cognitive biases was pioneered in the 1970s by psychologists Daniel Kahneman and Amos Tversky.[8] Kahneman was awarded the 2002 Nobel Prize for their work, and he later popularized these concepts with the general public in his best-selling 2011 book, *Thinking, Fast and Slow*.[3] The principles of their work have since been applied to decision making in numerous fields, including economics, professional sports, and medicine.[9,10]

Heuristics play a large and increasingly studied role in clinical decision making. In this setting, a clinician's previous experiences and personal perceptions (biases) guide decision making and create mental shortcuts (heuristics) to answer a clinical question or make a decision.[11] Heuristic decision making typically entails that the clinician focus on just a few salient features of a case or clinical question and ignore the remainder of available information.[12] In this way, experienced clinicians can make decisions accurately and more efficiently than by using more complex methods of decision making.[6,13]

The role of heuristics and cognitive biases deserves special attention in considering the nature of medical decision making and the causes of diagnostic error. Although definitions on diagnostic error vary, it has been demonstrated that the large majority of such errors are due to failures in clinician thinking and cognitive errors (rather than systems-based failures).[14,15] In one study, a cognitive error was found to be associated with diagnostic error in nearly 75% of cases.[15] Cognitive errors in medical decision making have thus been described as one of the major threats to patient safety.[16] Accordingly, there is significant incentive to understand the role of heuristics and bias in decision making and diagnostic quality.

HEALTHY HEURISTICS

Heuristics are simple, intuitive decision tools that are practical and effective in many clinical scenarios. They are guided by clinician experience and intuition, which refers to the ability to know something without analytical or conscious reasoning. They are used in much of the so-called flesh and blood decision making in medicine,[17] wherein clinicians "respond to omnipresent time pressures and resource availability with expeditious decision and action."[18]

Although this form of decision making has at times been portrayed as inferior, error-prone, or nonscientific, heuristics have rightfully been appreciated as powerful decision tools by many others.[19] Groopman[10] stresses the importance of heuristics, considering them to be "the foundation of all mature medical thinking." There are many features of heuristics that enable them to serve as valuable decision tools which function well in many clinical environments, especially fast-paced, high acuity settings.

Heuristics have many features that make them well suited for use in medical decision making. First, they are efficient and economical, allowing the clinician to make a good decision under significant time constraints.[11] This type of decision making is paramount in the ED or ICU, where decisions must often be made quickly and assertively to prevent loss of life or limb. For example, the clinician caring for a patient with a tension pneumothorax does not have the luxury of time to contemplate and analyze all aspects of the presentation. They must act urgently and instinctively, selectively ignoring other available information, to stabilize the patient. In scenarios such as these, heuristics typically serve clinicians well.

In addition, decisions made heuristically are effective in that they reduce the clinician's cognitive load, an important feature in settings with multiple competing priorities and high decision density. In the ED, for example, it has been estimated a clinician might make well over one thousand decisions in a single shift.[19] Productivity would drop precipitously and unsustainably if every single decision required methodical, deliberate type 2 analysis. In using heuristics, clinicians subconsciously reduce their cognitive load through use of shortcuts and intuitive reasoning instead of approaching every decision through an analytical method.[11]

As noted, although not infallible, heuristics are often accurate. This manner of thinking and decision making persists, in part, because it typically yields a positive result or correct diagnosis and provides positive reinforcement to the brain.[6] Heuristics are based on past experience and previous decisions, which have a track record of yielding the right answer and arriving at the correct conclusion. Numerous studies have demonstrated that, when used correctly, heuristics can outperform more sophisticated decision and prediction tools.[12,20]

For example, a heuristic was devised to aid clinicians in determining optimal disposition for adult patients with chest pain to either the cardiac ICU or general medicine unit. The simple tool outperformed a complicated logistic regression model with both greater sensitivity (proportion of patients correctly assigned to the cardiac ICU) and a lower false positive rate (proportion of patient incorrectly assigned to the cardiac ICU). The heuristic approach ignored selective information and considered only a fraction of information used by the regression model, yet it performed better while using fewer resources.[12]

To summarize, heuristics are powerful and integral decision tools that can aid the diagnostic process because they are efficient, often correct, and allow busy clinicians to make decisions and care for patients under time-constraints, competing priorities, and diagnostic uncertainty.

HEURISTIC FAILURES AND COGNITIVE BIASES

Despite their many positive attributes, heuristics are prone to failure. When heuristics fail, they are often labeled as cognitive errors or biases.[16] Crupi and Elia[21] note that cognitive error arises from "the spontaneous application of intuitive heuristic processes that are commonly triggered, largely effective, and inherent to the human mind." Cognitive biases are pervasive, universal, and inherent to human cognition and thus warrant further review.[6]

COGNITIVE DISPOSITIONS TO RESPOND

Although cognitive biases have been portrayed as inherently negative, it should be clarified that the term "bias" simply describes tendency of a person to respond to a situation in a particular manner or predictable way. In modern language, however, bias typically connotes negativity and may suggest prejudice (ie, gender or racial bias).[19] For this reason, some scholars favor the broader, less polarizing term "cognitive dispositions to respond" (CDR) to describe bias and promote a more objective approach to understanding their applications.[18,19] As with bias itself, CDRs are not considered errors in and of themselves. It is when CDRs result in misdiagnosis or adverse outcomes that they are described as cognitive errors.[19]

The psychology literature has described more than 100 different types of CDRs or cognitive biases, more than 30 of which are relevant to the practice of medical decision making and clinical diagnosis.[16,19,22] A select list of relevant biases is further described in **Table 2**. Among these, anchoring and availability biases are the most well studied, although premature closure is perhaps most common in clinical practice.[15,27–29] Given the complexity of human cognition, there is often significant overlap in features of many biases.

To better illustrate some of the more common biases, included here are some clinical examples based on actual case reports that highlight the role of cognitive bias in diagnosis and management.

Availability Bias

There have been increasing awareness and commercial publicity surrounding the recently described COVID-related multisystem inflammatory syndrome in children (MIS-C). The syndrome is rare but potentially life-threatening, and therefore, on the forefront of both parents' and clinicians' minds. A 3-year-old is admitted to the hospital with persistent fevers, and antibiotics are withheld while he is evaluated for MIS-C. Two days into his hospitalization, his urine culture returned positive for *Escherichia coli*, and subsequently, a renal ultrasound revealed renal scarring.[30]

In this unfortunate case, the clinicians were influenced by the recent prevalence and publicity of a newly described syndrome.[31] Because the MIS-C diagnosis was immediately available in their minds, the clinicians initially failed to manage other potential causes of the child's fever. Aware of their error, clinicians in this case will likely be vigilant about assessing and treating for pyelonephritis when they next encounter a child hospitalized for fever. In this way, the diagnoses made (or not made) influence subsequent decisions and the availability bias persists.

Triage Cueing and Anchoring Bias

During the COVID-19 pandemic, an ED triage nurse evaluates a young man with chief complaints of sore throat, fever, and chest pain. Despite having two negative COVID-19 tests as an outpatient within the prior seven days, he is triaged to the "COVID pod" in the ED, which cohorts patients suspected of having severe acute respiratory syndrome coronavirus 2 (SARS-CoV-2). His physical examination is notable for tachycardia, hypotension, exudative pharyngitis, and increasing respiratory distress. Workup demonstrates negative rapid testing for *Streptococcus pyogenes*, influenza, and Epstein-Barr virus. His chest radiograph reveals bilateral nodular densities with

Table 2
Cognitive biases and heuristics

Bias/Heuristic	Definition	Notes
Anchoring[19,23]	The tendency to focus on the first piece of information offered (the "anchor") and base the likelihood of the diagnosis on information available at the start. A "first impression bias"	Compounded by confirmation bias; may lead to premature closure
Availability[21,23,24]	The tendency to judge a diagnosis as being more likely or probable if it readily comes to mind; when a clinician has recently diagnosed a condition, they are more likely to seek out that diagnosis in the next similar patient encounter	Supported by the mantra "common things being common" and leads to overdiagnosis of common conditions
Ascertainment[19]	The clinician's thought process is influenced by what the clinician expects to find	Patient stereotyping and gender bias may be examples of ascertainment
Confirmation bias[11,21]	Accepting only evidence that confirms a diagnostic impression; rejecting evidence that is contradictory; "tunnel vision"	Closely aligned with anchoring, perpetuates premature closure
Diagnostic momentum[16,19]	A diagnostic label is assigned without adequate evidence and is then perpetuated across various settings and providers within the health care system	Results in an error due to inheriting someone else's thinking
Overconfidence bias[19,25]	Believing one knows more than one does; prioritizing opinion or authority rather than evidence	
Premature closure[16,23]	The tendency to stop too early in the diagnostic process, which concludes before the diagnosis has been fully verified. "When the diagnosis is made, the thinking stops"	Perpetuated by confirmation bias
Search satisficing[19,23]	The disposition to call off a search once something (abnormal) is found	Can perpetuate premature closure
Triage cueing[26]	Labels assigned in triage impact subsequent management and decision making	The phrase "Geography is destiny" embodies this notion
Unpacking principle[19]	Failing to explore data thoroughly, resulting in the failure to uncover important findings	For example: A clinician reviews the radiology report but not the actual image

a ground-glass appearance. He is admitted to the COVID unit of the ICU while his third COVID-19 test is pending (it also returned negative). Additional workup reveals a non-occlusive thrombus of his left interior jugular vein, and his blood cultures eventually grow *Fusobacterium* and group G streptococcus, consistent with Lemierre syndrome.[32]

This case demonstrates the several heuristic failures, starting with triage cueing. Labels and locations assigned by the triage nurse can strongly influence the course of management and subsequent decision making.[26] The phrase "geography is destiny" has been used to characterize this concept.[33] Furthermore, the medical team anchored on the patient's complaint of fever and chest pain and attributed these symptoms to SARS-CoV-2, when in fact they were the result of the bacterial infection and associated septic pulmonary microemboli known to occur in Lemierre syndrome. Finally, this case again demonstrates the availability bias: with a high prevalence of COVID-19 in this setting, clinicians assigned that diagnosis as most likely and proceeded as such.

Confirmation Bias and Premature Closure

It is January in the ICU, and a 36-year-old man with asthma, anxiety, and depression is admitted from the ED with a flulike illness. He has high fever, tachycardia, tachypnea, diarrhea, and malaise, but his symptoms have not responded to intravenous fluids or antipyretics. Curiously, the patient is noted to have new onset hypertension and significant agitation. His symptoms fail to improve with supportive care, and his mental status worsens. The ICU team later obtains additional history, reviews the patient's medication list, and repeats the physical examination, which demonstrates clonus. The patient is diagnosed with serotonin syndrome, and his symptoms improve once the offending agents are discontinued.[34,35]

This scenario demonstrates confirmation bias and premature closure. The patient presented during peak flu season with "fever" and malaise. He was presumed to have the flu, even though some of his symptoms, such as hypertension and altered mental status, were not consistent with this diagnosis. Had the team paid more attention to the patient's seemingly aberrant symptoms and considered all evidence, the accurate diagnosis might have been made more promptly. Accepting only evidence that confirms the diagnostic impression is confirmation bias. In addition, once admitted to the ICU, the working diagnosis was initially accepted without further workup or consideration. In this way, premature closure affected the team's ability to make the correct diagnosis in a timelier fashion.

Diagnostic Momentum

A 22-year-old woman presents with a long-standing history of abdominal pain and nausea with vomiting. She had been evaluated by her primary physician, and her chart notes her past medical history includes diagnoses of both anorexia nervosa and chronic abdominal pain. She has had multiple visits at different EDs for abdominal pain, where these diagnoses have not been questioned, and has had several admissions for electrolyte abnormalities. It is not until she presents in hypovolemic shock that a more extensive evaluation revealed a diagnosis of primary adrenal insufficiency.[36]

Here, a young woman was incorrectly diagnosed with anorexia nervosa, and once that diagnostic label was applied to the patient and her medical record, it was accepted at face value by subsequent clinicians in multiple settings. The diagnosis persisted across several different health settings and different clinicians, who fell victim to the diagnostic momentum bias. In the ICU setting, where most patients arrive with a diagnostic label,[7] clinicians must be sure to carefully and critically evaluate preestablished diagnoses and avoid this type of bias.

DETERMINANTS OF COGNITIVE DISPOSITIONS TO RESPOND

In considering bias and CDRs in clinical practice, it is helpful to understand the many factors that affect decision making and contribute to heuristic failure.

- *Ambient conditions*: The clinical setting, including its available resources, staffing, bed availability, patient volume, and support services, affect CDRs.[18]
- *Past experience*: Clinician experience begets expertise, and novice clinicians have fewer experiences from which to develop and refine heuristic thinking.[18]
- *Affective state*: The clinician's mood and disposition, which may vary throughout a shift, are affected by factors both internal and external to the clinical environment (social dynamics, personal health and temperament, circadian rhythms, risk-tolerance, other personality traits, and so forth).
- *Patient factors*: Patient behaviors or traits may elicit positive or negative responses from the clinician. Patient gender or race may influence decision making.[37,38] Finally, heuristic processes are more prone to failure when patient presentations are atypical.[5]
- *Team factors*: Rapport, cooperation, and interpersonal dynamics affect decision making and CDR. Delegation of the cognitive workload may facilitate reduction in the clinician's overall cognitive burden.[18]
- *Fatigue*: Sleep deprivation, sleep debt, and fatigue can adversely affect memory, reasoning, attention, and vigilance and impair cognitive performance, resulting in error.[39]

Many factors influence clinical decision making and can affect CDR. Some factors are modifiable, whereas many are largely out of a clinician's ability to control. Notably, the incidence of cognitive biases increases in uncertainty and when decision making is hurried or pressured.[40] In addition, the risk of diagnostic error and cognitive failure is greater in patients with complex presentations.[25] Understanding CDRs and the scenarios when they tend to occur may be one way to mitigate cognitive bias.

MITIGATING COGNITIVE BIAS

Given the potential for diagnostic failure and patient harm, a variety of strategies have been proposed to reduce and overcome biases. Some scholars have suggested that the most important strategy involves raising awareness through strategic student and clinician education. Clinicians must first be aware of the many existing cognitive biases or CDRs that are relevant to medical decision making in order to then understand how to avoid them.[41,42] Preliminary work has shown, however, that even after clinicians receive training in biases, they are not reliably able to identify them when present in the diagnostic process.[43] Others have questioned the notion that cognitive biases can be mitigated.[44] Nevertheless, cognitive debiasing strategies show potential for application in the diagnostic setting and continue to be investigated. Select strategies are summarized later and are reviewed in detail in a later article.

Metacognition

Simply put, metacognition means to think about thinking. It refers to one's ability to separate himself from his thoughts, evaluate his own thinking, and recognize opportunities for improvement.[40] Incumbent to this process is the ability to self-monitor and self-critique, as well as the skill to recognize one's limitations and identify strategies to manage diagnostic failure. This amounts to an intentional cognitive intervention during the reasoning process.[40]

Cognitive Forcing Strategies

These strategies comprise a specific debiasing technique wherein the clinician consciously and conscientiously self-monitors their decision making. A metacognitive step is intentionally inserted into the diagnostic process, and the clinician pauses their thought process to consider alternatives to diagnosis or potential pitfalls in their line of reasoning. These strategies have been subclassified as either generic or specific.[40]

With generic cognitive forcing strategies, the clinician possesses an understanding of the major classes of biases that affect decision making and thus uses a general rule to avoid error. In the acute care setting, one commonly used strategy is to "rule-out the worst-case scenario."[19] By embracing this mantra, emergency clinicians identify the life- or limb-threatening diagnoses associated with a given symptom or complaint and systematically rule out these conditions.

In specific cognitive forcing strategies, the clinician identifies a specific scenario in which errors are known to occur and applies the strategy to avoid the pitfall.[40] For example, a clinician evaluating a trauma patient with a seat-belt sign on the abdomen recalls that not only does this herald potential small bowel injury but also there is often an associated chance fracture of the lumbar spine. The clinician performs an examination and orders imaging to assess for both injuries with the awareness that the spinal fracture tends to initially be overlooked.

Although some preliminary work has suggested limited utility and even futility to cognitive forcing strategies,[45] many others support cognitive bias mitigation as an effective way to reduce error and potentially prevent patient harm.[46]

BIAS RESEARCH AND FUTURE DIRECTIONS

Importantly, recent research has worked to better quantify and describe the role of gestalt, heuristics, and bias in diagnostic error, although this work is in its infancy and requires further appraisal. Multiple recent studies have evaluated the accuracy of real-time clinician gestalt (often in comparison to a validated clinical decision aid or prediction rule), and results have been mixed. In a study assessing the risk of serious bacterial infection (SBI) in febrile infants, clinician suspicion was not reliable in identifying patients with SBIs.[47] Similar findings have been reported for clinician gestalt in ruling in or out acute coronary syndrome in adults presenting with chest pain.[48] Conversely, other work has validated the reliability of clinician gestalt in multiple clinical scenarios, including the prediction of appendicitis in children presenting with abdominal pain, the prediction of serious intra-abdominal injury in children with blunt torso trauma, the identification of adults with pulmonary embolism, and the diagnosis of adults with COVID-19.[49–53] A recent report noted that studies evaluating clinical decision aids rarely compare the performance of the decision aid to unaided clinician gestalt. Notably, in a sample of 21 studies that did compare a decision aid to clinician gestalt, only two studies found the aid to be superior to clinician judgment.[54] Ongoing work should characterize clinician gestalt in a variety of clinical settings and compare intuition to established decision aids. Finally, with the increasing potential to use artificial intelligence (AI) in diagnosis and clinical decision making, future work should compare AI to clinician gestalt.[55,56]

Bias is another topic of active investigation. Given the practical and ethical challenges of evaluating heuristics in actual medical decision-making scenarios, most of the research in cognitive bias is conducted through surveys, hypothetical vignettes, and simulated scenarios.[11,27,43] As such, it is lacking in generalizability and real-world application. Other criticisms of current research note that only a handful of biases have been studied (the availability bias being one of the more popular) and the tendency to study the decision in question in isolation, as single-decision event. Future work should therefore focus on high-quality investigation of actual decision making in its natural setting and across multiple medical disciplines.[28] Last, the scope of research should be broadened to study the full catalog of cognitive biases.[27] With better understanding of human cognition, heuristics, and biases, it is anticipated that strategies can be developed to optimize decision making, reduce cognitive errors, and improve patient care.

SUMMARY

Dual process theory describes human thinking in terms of two systems: one fast and automatic, the other slow and methodical. Heuristics, or mental shortcuts, are a key feature of system 1 or intuitive reasoning. Heuristics are applied instinctively and are often accurate, which is helpful when clinicians are working under suboptimal conditions (stress, fatigue, high decisional density) or are caring for multiple complicated patients simultaneously. Heuristics are also prone to failures, or cognitive biases, which can lead to diagnostic errors and patient harm. A variety of cognitive debiasing strategies have been proposed to mitigate heuristic failure; however, further investigation is required to optimize strategies and improve clinical diagnosis.

CLINICS CARE POINTS

- Heuristics are helpful rules of thumb or mental shortcuts that allow for decisions to be made efficiently and accurately under stress, time-constraints, high cognitive load, and large decision density.
- Heuristics often lead to accurate conclusions and correct diagnoses but can be prone to catastrophic failure.
- Failed heuristics are described as cognitive biases or cognitive dispositions to respond.
- Many cognitive biases relevant to the practice of medicine have been described, and ongoing research seeks to better understand their role in diagnosis and devise strategies to prevent cognitive error.

DISCLOSURE

C.W. Mangus has no disclosures or conflicts of interest. P. Mahajan has no disclosures or conflicts of interest.

REFERENCES

1. Croskerry P. A universal model of diagnostic reasoning. Acad Med 2009;84(8): 1022–8.
2. Evans JS. Dual-processing accounts of reasoning, judgment, and social cognition. Annu Rev Psychol 2008;59:255–78.
3. Kahneman D. Thinking, fast and slow. New York: Farrar, Straus, and Giroux; 2011.
4. Hammond K. Human judgment and social policy: irreducible uncertainty, inevitable error, unavoidable injustice. New York, NY: Oxford University Press; 2000.
5. McDonald CJ. Medical heuristics: the silent adjudicators of clinical practice. Ann Intern Med 1996;124(1 Pt 1):56–62.
6. Croskerry P. Bias: a normal operating characteristic of the diagnosing brain. Diagnosis (Berl) 2014;1(1):23–7.

7. Bergl PA, Nanchal RS, Singh H. Diagnostic error in the critically Ill: defining the problem and exploring next steps to advance intensive care unit safety. Ann Am Thorac Soc 2018;15(8):903–7.

8. Tversky A, Kahneman D. Judgment under uncertainty: heuristics and biases. Science 1981;211:453–8.

9. Lemire J. This book is not about baseball. But baseball teams swear by it. The New York Times; 2021. Available at: https://www.nytimes.com/2021/02/24/sports/baseball/thinking-fast-and-slow-book.html?smid=url-share. Accessed April 8, 2021.

10. Groopman J. How doctors think. New York, NY: Houghton Mifflin Company; 2007.

11. Whelehan DF, Conlon KC, Ridgway PF. Medicine and heuristics: cognitive biases and medical decision-making. Ir J Med Sci 2020;189(4):1477–84.

12. Marewski JN, Gigerenzer G. Heuristic decision making in medicine. Dialogues Clin Neurosci 2012;14(1):77–89.

13. Gigerenzer G, Gaissmaier W. Heuristic decision making. Annu Rev Psychol 2011; 62:451–82.

14. Weingart SN, Wilson RM, Gibberd RW, et al. Epidemiology of medical error. BMJ 2000;320:774–7.

15. Graber ML, Franklin N, Gordon R. Diagnostic error in internal medicine. Arch Intern Med 2005;165(13):1493–9.

16. Campbell SG, Croskerry P, Bond WF. Profiles in patient safety: a "perfect storm" in the emergency department. Acad Emerg Med 2007;14(8):743–9.

17. Reason J. Human error. New York: Cambridge University Press; 1990.

18. Croskerry P. Diagnostic failure: a cognitive and affective approach. In: Henriksen K, Battles JB, Marks ES, et al, editors. Advances in patient safety: from research to implementation (volume 2: concepts and methodology). Rockville (MD): Agency for Healthcare Research and Quality (US); 2005.

19. Croskerry P. Achieving quality in clinical decision making: cognitive strategies and detection of bias. Acad Emerg Med 2002;9(11):1184–204.

20. Gigerenzer G, Brighton H. Homo heuristicus: why biased minds make better inferences. Top Cogn Sci 2009;1(1):107–43.

21. Crupi V, Elia F. Understanding and improving decisions in clinical medicine (I): reasoning, heuristics, and error. Intern Emerg Med 2017;12:689–91.

22. Hughes TM, Dossett LA, Hawley ST, et al. Recognizing heuristics and bias in clinical decision-making. Ann Surg 2020;271(5):813–4.

23. Croskerry P. Cognitive and affective dispositions to respond. In: Croskerry P, Cosby K, Schenkel S, et al, editors. Patient safety in emergency medicine. Philadelphia, PA: Lippincott Williams & Wilkins; 2009. p. 219–27.

24. Mamede S, van Gog T, van den Berge K, et al. Effect of availability bias and reflective reasoning on diagnostic accuracy among internal medicine residents. JAMA 2010;304(11):1198–203.

25. Bordini BJ, Stephany A, Kliegman R. Overcoming diagnostic errors in medical practice. J Pediatr 2017;185:19–25.e1.

26. Croskerry P, Wears RL. Safety errors in emergency medicine. In: Markovchick VJ, Pons PT, editors. Emergency medicine secrets. 3rd edition. Philadelphia: Hanley and Belfus; 2003.

27. Blumenthal-Barby JS, Krieger H. Cognitive biases and heuristics in medical decision making: a critical review using a systematic search strategy. Med Decis Making 2015;35(4):539–57.

28. Saposnik G, Redelmeier D, Ruff CC, et al. Cognitive biases associated with medical decisions: a systematic review. BMC Med Inform Decis Mak 2016;16(1):138.

29. Schiff GD, Hasan O, Kim S, et al. Diagnostic error in medicine: analysis of 583 physician-reported errors. Arch Intern Med 2009;169:1881–7.
30. Molloy M, Jerardi K, Marshall T. What are we missing in our search for MIS-C? Hosp Pediatr 2021;11(4):e66–9.
31. Schmidt HG, Mamede S, van den Berge K, et al. Exposure to media information about a disease can cause doctors to misdiagnose similar-looking clinical cases. Acad Med 2014;89(2):285–91.
32. Karn MN, Johnson NP, Yaeger SK, et al. A teenager with fever, chest pain, and respiratory distress during the coronavirus disease 2019 pandemic: a lesson on anchoring bias. J Am Coll Emerg Physicians Open 2020;1(6):1392–4.
33. Perry SJ. Profiles in patient safety: organizational barriers to patient safety. Acad Emerg Med 2002;9(8):848–50.
34. Jindal S, Gombar S, Jain K. Serotonin syndrome in ICU-a road less traveled. Indian J Crit Care Med 2019;23(8):376–7.
35. Navarroza RV, Zamora LD, Navarra SV. Serotonin syndrome masquerading as disease flare in lupus nephritis with end-stage renal disease. Int J Rheum Dis 2019;22(10):1933–6.
36. Feeney C, Buell K. A case of Addison's disease nearly mistaken for anorexia nervosa. Am J Med 2018;131(11):e457–8.
37. Raine R. Bias measuring bias. J Health Serv Res Policy 2002;7:65–7.
38. Schulman KA, Berlin JA, Harless W, et al. The effect of race and sex on physician's recommendations for cardiac catheterization. NEJM 1999;340:618–26.
39. Bonnet MH. Sleep deprivation. In: Kryger M, Roth T, Dement WC, editors. Principles and practice of sleep medicine. Philadelphia: Saunders; 2000. p. 53–71.
40. Croskerry P. Cognitive forcing strategies in clinical decisionmaking. Ann Emerg Med 2003;41(1):110–20.
41. Croskerry P. The importance of cognitive errors in diagnosis and strategies to minimize them. Acad Med 2003;78(8):775–80.
42. Ryan A, Duignan S, Kenny D, et al. Decision making in paediatric cardiology. Are we prone to heuristics, biases and traps? Pediatr Cardiol 2018;39(1):160–7.
43. Zwaan L, Monteiro S, Sherbino J, et al. Is bias in the eye of the beholder? A vignette study to assess recognition of cognitive biases in clinical case workups. BMJ Qual Saf 2017;26(2):104–10.
44. Klein GA, Orasanu J, Calderwood R, et al, editors. Decision making in action: models and methods. Norwood, NJ: Ablex Publishing; 1995.
45. Sherbino J, Kulasegaram K, Howey E, et al. Ineffectiveness of cognitive forcing strategies to reduce biases in diagnostic reasoning: a controlled trial. CJEM 2014;16(1):34–40.
46. Lambe KA, O'Reilly G, Kelly BD, et al. Dual-process cognitive interventions to enhance diagnostic reasoning: a systematic review. BMJ Qual Saf 2016;25: 808–20.
47. Nigrovic LE, Mahajan PV, Blumberg SM, et al. Febrile Infant Working Group of the Pediatric Emergency Care Applied Research Network (PECARN). The Yale Observation Scale score and the risk of serious bacterial infections in febrile infants. Pediatrics 2017;140(1):e20170695.
48. Oliver G, Reynard C, Morris N, et al. Can emergency physician gestalt "rule in" or "rule out" acute coronary syndrome: validation in a multicenter prospective diagnostic cohort study. Acad Emerg Med 2020;27(1):24–30.
49. Lee WH, O'Brien S, Skarin D, et al. Accuracy of clinician gestalt in diagnosing appendicitis in children presenting to the emergency department. Emerg Med Australas 2019;31(4):612–8.

50. Simon LE, Kene MV, Warton EM, et al. Diagnostic performance of emergency physician gestalt for predicting acute appendicitis in patients age 5 to 20 years. Acad Emerg Med 2020;27(9):821–31.
51. Mahajan P, Kuppermann N, Tunik M, et al. Intra-abdominal Injury Study Group of the Pediatric Emergency Care Applied Research Network (PECARN). Comparison of clinician suspicion versus a clinical prediction rule in identifying children at risk for intra-abdominal injuries after blunt torso trauma. Acad Emerg Med 2015;22(9):1034–41.
52. Penaloza A, Verschuren F, Meyer G, et al. Comparison of the unstructured clinician gestalt, the Wells score, and the revised Geneva score to estimate pretest probability for suspected pulmonary embolism. Ann Emerg Med 2013;62(2): 117–24.e2.
53. Nazerian P, Morello F, Prota A, et al. Diagnostic accuracy of physician's gestalt in suspected COVID-19: prospective bicentric study. Acad Emerg Med 2021;28(4): 404–11.
54. Schriger DL, Elder JW, Cooper RJ. Structured clinical decision aids are seldom compared with subjective physician judgment and are seldom superior. Ann Emerg Med 2017;70(3):338–44.e3.
55. Kirubarajan A, Taher A, Khan S, et al. Artificial intelligence in emergency medicine: a scoping review. J Am Coll Emerg Physicians Open 2020;1(6):1691–702.
56. Krittanawong C. The rise of artificial intelligence and the uncertain future for physicians. Eur J Intern Med 2018;48:e13–4.

Enhancing Analytical Reasoning in the Intensive Care Unit

Mark Barash, DO, Rahul S. Nanchal, MD, MS*

KEYWORDS

- Bayes theorem • Bias • Clinical reasoning • Heuristics • Logic • Noise • Probability
- Set theory • Venn diagrams

KEY POINTS

- Intensivists often rely on heuristic principles that lead to severe and systematic errors in reasoning.
- Reasoning foundations can be described mathematically using logic, probability, and value theory.
- Intensivists should familiarize themselves with basic statistical and probability principles to enhance analytical reasoning and avoid biases.
- Bayesian reasoning is the framework surrounding the calculation of posterior odds of events.
- Noise is likely pervasive in the intensive care unit and should be mitigated.

INTRODUCTION

Clinical reasoning in critical care presents numerous challenges because decisions must be made expeditiously. Further, there is considerable uncertainty associated with the decision-making process due to patient complexity, severity of illness, and the enormous array of laboratory values and physiologic parameters that require distillation into a diagnosis that is most compatible with the clinical presentation. The cognitive load associated with these complexities combined with situational stressors of time-sensitive conditions and rapidly deteriorating patients leads to reliance on heuristic principles that reduce the intricate tasks of assessing probabilities and assigning predictive values to simpler judgmental operations. Although useful, these heuristics often lead to severe and systematic errors of reasoning.[1] Decision making or judgment encompasses processes that are amenable to systemic analysis in addition to those that are intangible and value decisions.

Division of Pulmonary and Critical Care Medicine, Hub for Collaborative Medicine, Medical College of Wisconsin, 8701 Watertown Plank Road, 8th Floor, Milwaukee, WI 53226, USA
* Corresponding author.
E-mail address: rnanchal@mcw.edu

Crit Care Clin 38 (2022) 51–67
https://doi.org/10.1016/j.ccc.2021.09.001
0749-0704/22/© 2021 Elsevier Inc. All rights reserved.

Reasoning foundations can be described mathematically using probability, symbolic logic, and value theory.[2] Intuitive—but ultimately misguided—judgment of these mathematical concepts is what leads to systematic errors. The components of error comprise biases and the emerging concept of noise. In this article, we first describe common errors in judgment due to cognitive biases and the mathematical basis underpinning them. We then describe mathematical concepts with which intensivists should be acquainted to minimize reasoning errors. We cite examples to illustrate concepts whereby appropriate. Finally, we end with a brief discussion of noise and its pertinence to critical care medicine.

ERRORS IN JUDGMENT AND MATHEMATICAL UNDERPINNINGS

A comprehensive list of heuristics and biases with brief descriptions appears in **Table 1**. We explain in detail a select few that are encountered most often in clinical practice. Problems in probabilistic and statistical reasoning are the mathematical underpinning for most of these biases.

Base rate neglect

Simply stated, base rate neglect is the failure to correctly account for the probability of a condition or disease which may lead to consequences such as unnecessary and expensive tests, faulty diagnoses, and inappropriate therapies. Providers often overlook that uncommon presentations of common diseases are more likely than common presentations of rare disorders. For example, an immigrant from a region with endemic tuberculosis presenting with multiple organ failure and laboratory features consistent with primary hemophagocytic lymphohistiocytosis (HLH) is far more likely to have disseminated tuberculosis than primary HLH.

Perhaps the most widespread form of base rate neglect is insensitivity to prior probabilities and anchoring bias to new but incomplete information that frequently becomes available in the context of critical illness. Consider an instance whereby laboratory tests are obtained on an elderly woman presenting with confusion and fever. Findings of anemia and thrombocytopenia may prompt an evaluation of thrombotic thrombocytopenic purpura (TTP). However, the prior probability of sepsis is manifold higher than TTP, and even with the new information of anemia and thrombocytopenia, the posterior probability of sepsis remains much larger than TTP. It would be an error not to evaluate for sepsis and administer antibiotics. Further, even when explicitly presented with base rate information, people often display ineptness and ignore the information. An adaptation of a well-known test is as follows: Leptospirosis as a cause of sepsis occurs at a frequency of 1 in 1000. A middle-aged man presents with sepsis; the source is undifferentiated. He is quickly intubated for respiratory distress and multiple organ failure ensues. Further history is not obtainable. Among the array of investigations that are performed, the test for leptospirosis is positive. The false-negative rate of the test is zero and the false-positive rate is 5%. What is the probability that this particular patient has leptospirosis? Most physicians would answer 95% simply taking into account that the test has a 95% accuracy rate. The correct answer is the conditional probability that the patient is sick and the test is positive which is less than 2%. A simple approach to arrive at the answer uses frequencies. Out of 1000 patients with similar presentations and testing regardless of whether they are suspected of having leptospirosis, only one is expected to have the disease. Out of the 999 that do not have the disease 5% or approximately 50 will have a positive test (because the false positive rate is 5%). Thus, the probability of having the disease for someone who has a positive test should be the ratio of the

Table 1
Heuristics

Heuristic/Bias	Description	Consequences
Aggregate bias	Associations between variables representing group averages are mistakenly taken to reflect what is true for a particular individual, usually when the individual measures are not available. An individual patient may be treated differently from what has been agreed upon through clinical practice guidelines for a group of patients (there is a tendency for some physicians to treat their own patients as atypical).	Physician noncompliance in idiosyncratic approaches may result in patients receiving tests, procedures, and treatment outside of accepted clinical practice guidelines.
Anchoring	A tendency to fixate on specific features of a presentation too early in the diagnostic process. The likelihood of a particular event is based on information at the outset. Some clinicians may fail to adjust their impressions based on new information as it arrives.	Anchoring may lead to premature closure of thinking leading to an incorrect diagnosis early in the patient's presentation.
Ascertainment bias	The physician's thinking is pre-shaped by expectations or by what the physician specifically hopes to find. A physician may be dismissive of abdominal pain in a patient who is admitted frequently for diabetic ketoacidosis. Stereotyping and gender biases are examples of ascertainment biases.	Any prejudgment of patients may lead to under-assessing or over-assessing a condition.
Availability and non- availability	The tendency to diagnose a condition more frequently if it comes more readily to mind. In other words, things that are common will be readily recalled. Nonavailability occurs when insufficient attention is paid to what is not immediately present.	Availability and non-availability lead to disproportionate estimates of the frequency of a particular diagnosis or condition, to starting estimates of the base rate, thus influencing pretest probability.

(continued on next page)

Table 1
(continued)

Heuristic/Bias	Description	Consequences
Base rate neglect	Failure to adequately take into account the prevalence of a particular disease.	May result in over-estimates of unlikely diagnoses. This may lead to wastefulness and over utilization of resources. The pursuit of esoteric diagnosis is occasionally successful, and the intermittent reinforcement sustains this behavior in some physicians.
Commission bias	Tendency toward action rather than inaction. This may occur in someone who is overconfident and reflects an urge to "do something."	Commission errors tend to change the course of events, because they involve an active intervention, and may therefore be less reversible than an error of omission.
Confirmation bias	A tendency to look for confirming evidence to support the hypothesis, rather than look for disconfirming evidence to refute it.	Confirmation bias leads to the preservation of hypotheses and diagnoses that were weak in the first place.
Diagnostic momentum	Tendency for a particular diagnosis to become established without adequate evidence. This may involve several intermediaries including the patient and other health care providers. As this is passed from person to person, the diagnosis gathers momentum to the point that it may appear almost certain by the time that the patient sees a physician.	A diagnosis may gather momentum without gathering verification. Delayed or missed diagnoses lead to the highest disabilities and are the most costly.

Term	Description	
Fundamental attribution error	The tendency to blame people when things go wrong rather than circumstances.	Reflects a lack of compassion and understanding for certain classes of patient and may result in inappropriate or compromised care.
Hindsight bias	After an event has occurred, there is a tendency to exaggerate the likelihood that would have been assessed for the event before it occurred. This may distort the perception of previous decision making, such as occurs at morbidity mortality rounds.	May prevent a realistic appraisal of what actually occurred and compromise learning from the event. It may lead to both under- and over-estimations of the clinical decision maker's abilities.
Omission bias	A tendency toward inaction or reluctance to treat.	While inaction may often be the most appropriate course, omission bias may result in the development of worsening. Emergencies.
Outcome bias	The tendency to judge the decision being made by its likely outcome. Physicians may prefer decisions that lead to good outcomes rather than those that lead to bad outcomes.	Allowing Personal hopes and desires to enter clinical decision making reduces objectivity and may significantly compromise the process.
Playing the odds	A physician's opinion of the relative chances that a patient has a particular disease or not. It is influenced by the actual prevalence and incidence of the disease. The decision is primarily determined by inductive thinking rather than objective evidence that has ruled out the disease.	Playing the odds runs the risk of important conditions being missed.
Posterior probability error	A physician bases their estimate of the likelihood of disease on what has gone before. A patient may have several admissions with sepsis related to urinary tract infection; to make the assumption that the current admission is related to a urinary tract infection is an example of a posterior probability error.	This error may result in a wrong diagnosis being perpetrated or a new diagnosis being missed.
Premature closure	Physicians typically generate several diagnoses early in their encounter with a clinical problem. Premature closure occurs when one of these diagnoses is accepted before it has been fully verified.	Premature closure tends to stop further thinking.

Adapted from Croskerry P. Achieving quality in clinical decision making: cognitive strategies and detection of bias. Acad Emerg Med. 2002;9(11):1184-1204. https://doi.org/10.1111/j.1553-2712.2002.tb01574.x; with permission

number of people who have the disease to the number of true and false positive tests which here is 1 in 51. The approach of indiscriminate testing (ie, casting a wide net without sound hypotheses hoping that some test will return positive and will, in turn, lead to a diagnosis), which is commonly described as a "shotgun approach to medicine," more often than not is a setup for diagnostic error and downstream administration of inappropriate therapies and iatrogenic harm. The process of deriving posterior or conditional probabilities, commonly known as the Bayesian approach is useful in interpreting test results. This approach is described in some detail later in discussion in the mathematical concepts section.

Insensitivity to sample size

This bias results from the inability to account for sample size when evaluating probabilities from small samples drawn from a larger population. Sampling theory dictates that the probability of deviating from the population average is much higher in smaller samples just by random chance. This phenomenon is particularly true for critical illness, whereby the sample for any given disease or syndrome is derived from a much larger universe of persons who are hospitalized or treated as outpatients. Combined with the fact that ICU patients on average represent a far sicker population than their counterparts hospitalized on medical wards or treated as outpatients, posterior probabilities of encountering rare diagnoses are greater in the ICU than in other areas. The label of ICU physicians being great diagnosticians may have more to do with the odds of encountering uncommon diseases and the happenstance of diagnosis rather than cognitive ability.

   To illustrate, first consider the example of spontaneous intracranial hemorrhage (ICH) in patients without coagulopathy or thrombocytopenia. For any given probability of ICH, one is more likely to find higher rates in the ICU than the rest of the hospital based on sample size alone. This is akin to the higher probability of getting 100% heads with 3 fair coin tosses (probability = 1/8) than with 5 tosses (probability = 1/32). Using the same logic, it is also more likely to find the lowest rates of ICH in the ICU (the probability of not getting a single head is more if a fair coin is tossed thrice instead of 5 times). Relatively rare events causing such discrepancies may often be the target of intense scrutiny and quality improvement efforts, one example being the prevention of catheter-associated central line infections (CLABSIs); variations of CLABSI across ICUs in the same hospital may be nothing but phenomena of random chance. Mathematically, this represents De Moivre's equation[3] which states that the standard error of the mean is inversely proportional to the square root of the sample size.

   Illuminating this concept further, now consider an adverse drug reaction, daptomycin-associated eosinophilic pneumonia. For the sake of clarity, let us assume that 20% of patients receiving daptomycin develop this reaction. The use of daptomycin is likely more frequent in the ICU; hence for simplicity, let us also assume that the probability of daptomycin use in the ICU than in general medical wards is 80% to 20%. The posterior odds that 4 out of 5 consecutive patients who receive daptomycin and develop eosinophilic pneumonia in the ICU than a general ward are 224:1. Even if the diagnostic accuracy in the ICU was 50%, the odds of diagnosing cases would overwhelmingly be in the favor of the ICU physician. Asked an alternate way, given the same circumstances which would afford more diagnostic confidence: A working diagnosis of eosinophilic pneumonia in 4 out of 5 consecutive patients who received daptomycin in the ICU or a diagnosis in 10 out of consecutive 20 patients who received daptomycin on the floor? At first glance, the rate of diagnosis in the ICU (80%) far exceeds the rate on the ward (50%), which, given our hypothetical rate of 20%, seems highly improbable. However, closer scrutiny reveals that the probability of developing daptomycin-related eosinophilic pneumonia in 4 out of 5 patients in the ICU is orders of magnitude higher than 10 out of 20 patients on the floor. Accurate diagnosis with such a low probability of occurrence on the ward is quite the feat.

Misconception of regression

If 2 variables X and Y have the same distribution and the average X score for a group of selected individuals deviates from the mean of X by k units, then the average of their Y score usually will deviate from Y by less than k units. This phenomenon called regression toward the mean occurs frequently in everyday life and was described by Galton more than 150 years ago.[4] Let us return to the example of CLABSI. Mere observation will clarify that a particularly outstanding period of performance on the occurrence of CLABSI will inevitably be followed by a period whereby the performance was worse than the preceding period and vice-versa. Often this prompts extensive critical quality reviews during the period when performance deviated from organizational goals (often set at zero infections!) and accolades when performance exceeds them. This schema of administering rewards and admonishments is widespread and may lead to misperceptions about their effectiveness when changes are most likely to occur secondary to regression alone.

Fallacies of conjunctive and disjunctive events

These biases, particularly common in medicine are the consequence of anchoring. Psychological studies[5,6] indicate that people tend to overestimate the probability of conjunctive events and underestimate the probability of disjunctive events. An example of a conjunction fallacy occurs when a trainee alleges sepsis from pneumonia and urinary tract infection (UTI) when asked for a diagnosis. Even if the probability of pneumonia and UTI are individually high, the probability of them occurring together is quite low—that is, the overall probability of a conjunctive event is lower than the probability of each elementary event. This phenomenon is a simple explanation behind Occam's razor or the parsimony in diagnosis. Of course, deviations from this principle are bound to occur. A patient may have both pneumonia and UTI at the same time; it is possible but less probable. In the same vein, a trainee's judgment that the cause of sepsis is more likely from pneumonia rather than pneumonia or UTI constitutes a disjunction fallacy. Although the likelihood of pneumonia may be high, the likelihood or either pneumonia or UTI is higher than the probability of each elementary event. Biases in the evaluation of compound events are pervasive and influence a myriad of actions such as administration of therapies (eg, choice of antibiotics) and obtaining laboratory/imaging studies which have numerous downstream influences on iatrogenic harm (eg, *Clostridium difficile* colitis), costs of care as well as patient safety and quality.

MATHEMATICAL CONCEPTS
Set theory/Venn diagrams/logic concepts

Set theory is a branch of mathematical logic that pertains to the study of sets or collection of objects. Probability theory uses the language of sets which can be illustrated in the form of Venn diagrams. Probability is nothing but a scientific method of measuring uncertainty or quantifying randomness. Basic operations of sets include intersection, union, difference, and symmetric difference (**Fig. 1**).

Probability concepts

Probabilistic reasoning asks a clinician to answer 2 basic questions: (1) how representative is the patient's presentation of known disease and (2) what is the likelihood of

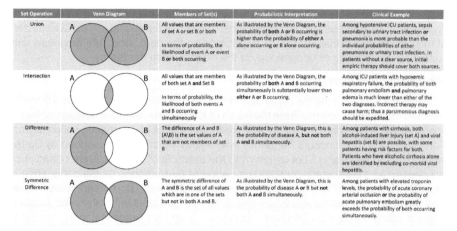

Fig. 1. Basic operations of sets.

encountering that disease in a patient like this?[7] The skilled diagnostician—whether formally or intuitively—may utilize a pretest probability based on historical and patient facts and determine the posttest probability, through a likelihood ratio that the disorder is indeed present. This approach is termed Bayesian reasoning. Before discussing Bayesian reasoning, we present concepts that intensivists must familiarize themselves with and are particularly useful in the interpretation of diagnostic test properties. These concepts illustrated in the form of 2 × 2 tables appear in **Fig. 2.**

Sensitivity

The proportion of true positives among those that have the disorder.

Specificity

The proportion of true negatives among those who do not have the disorder.

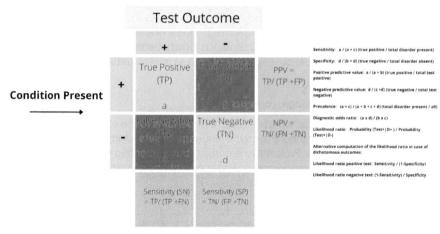

Fig. 2. Graphical representation and calculation of properties of diagnostics tests.

Predictive values

The absolute probability that the disorder is present or absent. It is important to note that predictive values depend on both test characteristics and the prevalence of the disorder. For example, an early warning system that has a sensitivity and specificity of 99% will have a positive predictive value of only 33% if the prevalence of clinical deterioration is 5 out of 1000 admissions. In other words, for every 100 alerts, on average, 67 will be false positive.

Likelihood ratios

The probability that a specific result is obtained in patient with the condition is divided by the probability that the same result is obtained in patients without the condition. A theoretic advantage of likelihood ratios is that they are independent of prevalence. In case of dichotomous measures, the likelihood ratio for a positive result can be calculated as sensitivity/1-specificity and the likelihood ratio for a negative result as 1-sensitivity/specificity.

Bayes theorem/reasoning

In 1736, Reverend Thomas Bayes (b. 1701) anonymously published "*An introduction to the doctrine of fluxions: and a defense of mathematicians against the objections of the author of the analyst.*"[8] In it were the first echoes of what, many years later, would be translated and reworked into Bayes theorem.

For epistemic rationality, probability estimates need to follow rules of objective probability. The most important of these are as follows: (a) Probabilities always vary between 0 and 1, (b) if an event is certain to happen, its probability is 1.0, (c) if an event is certain not to happen, then its probability is 0, and (d) if 2 events cannot both happen, then they are mutually exclusive and the probability of one OR the other occurring is the probability of each added together.

An important concept is that of conditional probability. Conditional probabilities concern the probability of an event A given that another event B has occurred. If A and B were mutually exclusive, then the probability of A occurring given that B has occurred would be zero. Thus, conditional probabilities usually deal with events that are not mutually exclusive. (A simple example of mutually exclusive events is the diagnosis of cholecystitis in someone who presents with fever, jaundice, and right upper quadrant pain but has previously undergone a cholecystectomy. Given that cholecystectomy has occurred, the probability of cholecystitis is zero.) Bayes theorem describes the probability of an event occurring while using knowledge about the local prevalence or risk factors of the condition itself. These represent the post and pretest probabilities, respectively. Mathematically, the Bayes theorem is represented via the formula.

$$P(A|B) = \frac{P(A)P(B|A)}{P(A)P(B|A)+P(\neg A)P(B|\neg A)}$$

where P(A|B) describes the likelihood of A occurring given B is true, P(B|A) describes the likelihood of B occurring given A is true, P(A) describes the probability of A occurring, P(B) describes the probability of B occurring and P(¬A) describes the probability of A not occurring which just 1 – the probability of A occurring. For judgment and decision making, the Bayes theorem has special importance because it allows a formal framework of updating beliefs in a hypothesis given new evidence. In clinical practice, it can be stated as posttest odds = pretest odds X likelihood ratio. Arriving at, and being confident in these values, is the crux of Bayesian reasoning.

Using the sensitivity and specificity of a test, a likelihood ratio (LR) is calculated and poses the question "what is the likelihood this patient has disease 'X' if presenting with complaint or test 'Y'." **Table 2** defines general values for LRs and their approximate effect on changing the posttest probability. **Fig. 3** shows a conversion graph for determining likelihood ratios from the sensitivity and specificity of positive and negative test results.

There is the tremendous utility of Bayesian reasoning in the critical care environment wherein patients often present with a gamut of complex problems, physical examination findings, historical features, and laboratory/imaging investigations. Instead of asking the clinician to consider the full range of differential diagnoses for a particular set of data, Bayesian reasoning ask the clinician to determine which is most likely based on the aforementioned information. Mathematically, if there is a hypothesis (H) and a set of collected data elements (D) then $P(H|D) = \frac{P(H) * P(H|D)}{P(H) * P(D|H) + p(\sim H) * P(D|\sim H)}$ where P(H) is the probability of the hypothesis _prior_ to collecting the data and (P ∼ H) is the probability that some alternate hypothesis is true before collecting the data. It is important to note that P(∼H) may represent any number of different hypotheses and that P(H) + P(∼H) may not equal 1.0. P(H|D) is the probability of hypothesis after the observed data pattern (posterior probability). Similarly, P(D|H) is the posterior probability of data given the hypothesis and P(D| ∼H) the posterior probability of data given alternative hypotheses. Here it is important to realize that P(D|H) and P(D| ∼H) are not complements and may not add up to 1.0. An illustrative example is an elderly patient presenting to the ICU with hypotension and altered mental status whereby the initial probabilities of septic shock and cardiogenic shock may be assigned probabilities of 0.5 and 0.2, given that from prior experience 50% and 20% of such patients presented with septic or cardiogenic shock, respectively. After physician examination reveals cool extremities, delayed capillary refill, and echocardiogram reveals a wall motion abnormality with depressed ejection fraction a clinician may judge that given these findings, the probability of cardiogenic shock is 0.6 and septic shock is 0.2. Thus, the posterior probabilities of cardiogenic and septic shock would be calculated as 0.54 and 0.45, respectively.

An important question revolves around clinician estimates of pretest probabilities. Judgment relies on several factors including the knowledge of the epidemiology of

Table 2 Approximate values for calculated likelihood ratios	
Likelihood Ratio	Approximate Change in Probability
Positive likelihood ratio value (+LR)	
1	+0%
2	+15%
5	+30%
10	+45%
Negative Likelihood ratio value (LR)	
0.1	−45%
0.2	−30%
0.5	−15%
1	−0%

Positive test result
Panel A

Negative test result
Panel B

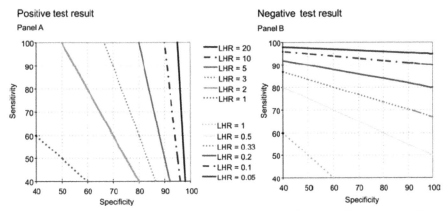

Fig. 3. Conversion graph for determining likelihood ratio from sensitivity and specificity. (*Adapted from* Fischer JE, Bachmann LM, Jaeschke R. A readers' guide to the interpretation of diagnostic test properties: clinical example of sepsis. Intensive Care Med. 2003;29(7):1043-1051. https://doi.org/10.1007/s00134-003-1761-8; with permission.)

the suspected disorder, utilization of risk calculators, or other validated analyses and clinical gestalt. Of course, the time available for decision making may influence one's ability to apply these concepts. An applicable scenario is that of a middle-aged female who presents with fevers, hypoxemia, cough with expectoration of dark phlegm, and a dense right basilar infiltrate on CT imaging. A plausible hypothesis may be pulmonary blastomycosis. If using basic epidemiology alone, someone practicing in the south-western USA might conclude that the likelihood is low and forgo additional investigation. Another clinician, practicing in a rural town in the upper Midwest, whereby blastomycosis is known to be hyperendemic, may conclude the pretest probability is high enough to either test via urinary antigen or, to even treat empirically while testing is pending. Risk calculators such as the PERC score[9] (for ruling out pulmonary embolism (PE)), LRINEC score[10] (for diagnosing necrotizing soft tissue infection), and PLASMIC score[11] (for predicting ADAMTS13 deficiency in thrombotic thrombocytopenia purpura) are just a few examples of readily available tools that may help a clinician, in the right circumstances, increase or decrease the likelihood that a disorder exists. As with all categorical variables, however, it is vital to understand the population in which these tests were developed and the limitations of the test. The PLASMIC score, for example, may only be used in a patient that already has thrombocytopenia and evidence of microangiopathic hemolytic anemia to *then* determine the probability that TTP exists.

In clinical practice and at the bedside, it is common for clinicians to use medical gestalt in estimating the pretest probability of a disorder, but limitations and failures exist. First, it should be noted that any estimate of the pretest probability of the disease will be a function of that clinician's biases and prior experience with such cases, knowledge about the presentation of the disease state and understanding of the utility of a certain complaint or examination findings as increasing or decreasing the likelihood of the disease existing. A wide variability in clinicians' assessment of pretest probability exists, adding to the lack of standardization. For example, Kline[12] evaluated clinician gestalt in estimating pretest probability for acute coronary syndrome (ACS) or PE in patients presenting with chest pain and dyspnea. Not surprisingly, clinicians significantly overestimated the presence of ACS (17% vs 4%; $P < .001$) and PE (12% vs 6%; $P < .01$) when compared with a validated computerized method. On the other hand, Penaloza[13] and colleagues performed a retrospective analysis of a prospective observational cohort of consecutive PE patients and compared gestalt with the Wells score and revised Geneva score. Clinicians (using gestalt) were more likely to label patients as either having "low" or "high" clinical probability of PE and the prevalence of PE was significantly lower with gestalt in low clinical probability groups. Likewise, gestalt better identified PE in nonhigh probability groups (low-medium probability).

Numerous biases can affect one's estimate of the pretest probability, as previously mentioned in **Table 1**. A common bias is anchoring which is the tendency to fixate on certain features of a case (ie, the first impression) and commonly leads to confirmation bias whereby the clinician then looks for—and places emphasis on—evidence to confirm their initial diagnosis. For example, a clinician may assume a patient with recurrent UTIs has a toxic encephalopathy related to a recurrent UTI, assuming elevated transaminase are the result of cholestasis of sepsis, while in fact disregarding the presence of palmar erythema, spider nevi, and palpable liver with international normalized ratio (INR) elevation suggestive of decompensated cirrhosis. This is also an example of a posterior probability error that perpetuates a previous diagnosis in a given patient. Some authors have argued that a pitfall of the probabilistic approach is that, by nature of its governing rules, it leads the clinician to disregard less common disease processes as evidenced by their low societal prevalence and therefore low pretest probability by proxy.[14] Thus, the Bayesian approach may accurately predict the likelihood of the disease in the broader population, but may fail to put the individual patient, with their idiosyncrasies, into context. In other words, Bayesian reasoning may provide the probability of a disease, but not necessarily the right answer. Bayesian approach to diagnosis also assumes that values for sensitivity and specificity are fixed. These values change with the evolution of the disease process. For instance, in the diagnosis of eosinophilia with granulomatosis and polyangiitis (EGPA), fixed or migratory pulmonary infiltrates carry a sensitivity and specificity of 15% to 30% and 92% to 94%, respectively.[15] However, EGPA is a triphasic disease with variable presentations and natural history that may take years to present with classical findings. Although pulmonary infiltrates are a diagnostic criterion, in the initial prodromic phase, this manifestation is generally absent and may lead a clinician to disregard the diagnosis outright.

Value theory concepts

After a diagnosis has been established clinicians must decide on appropriate treatment. Often this is relatively simple that is, administering available scientifically sound therapies that are standard for a diagnosis (eg, antibiotics for pneumonia). However, the choice of therapy frequently involves complex considerations that encompass therapeutic (benefit vs harm), ethical, moral, social, and economic dilemmas spanning patients, families, and society. A mathematic approach to these "value problems" is defined by value theory. One form of this approach is described by the threshold approach to treatment. In this approach, the clinician may (1) withhold further testing and treatment, (2) administer empiric therapy, and (3) perform additional testing and decide on therapy based on the results of this test[16] The choices are driven by a "testing threshold"—the probability of disease at which there is no difference in the value of withholding treatment and performing further testing and a "test-treatment threshold"—the probability of disease at which there is no difference between performing further testing and administering treatment. Calculations of these thresholds involve the assimilation of data describing risks and benefits of treatment and the risks of testing and tests characteristics indicating reliability. Treatment is withheld if the probability of disease is below the testing threshold and given if it is greater than the test-treatment threshold. Additional testing is performed if the probability lies between these 2 thresholds with treatment contingent on the results of the test. An excellent visual and mathematical review of this concept can be viewed in reference number 9.

A related approach uses game theory first developed by Von Neumann.[17] Game theory is the study of interactions between individuals by applying mathematical models of conflict and cooperation. These concepts may be applied to understand the complexities of treatments in the context of a variety of provider, patient, and family uncertainties.

Regardless of the approach, an important concept in value theory is that of the "expected value." To illustrate this concept, let us assume that a particular patient has one of the 2 diagnoses D1 and D2 with probabilities of 3/5 and 2/5, respectively. Let us also assume that there are 2 treatments T1 and T2. T1 is 80% effective for diagnosis D1 and 30% effective for diagnosis D2. Similarly, T2 is 20% effective for diagnosis D1 and 90% effective for diagnosis D2. The expected value of treatment T1 is $3/5 \times 80/100 + 2/5 \times 30/100$ which is equal to 60/100. The expected value of treatment T2 is $3/5 \times 20/100 + 2/5 \times 90/100$ which is equal to 48/100. In other words, given the same circumstances, 60 out of 100 patients would receive effective treatment if T1 were used as opposed to 48 out of 100 if T2 were used; hence T1 should be the preferred therapy. Assignment of treatment values may often require consideration of intangibles such as moral and ethical standards which require physician judgment. Values may be negative in cases whereby treatment may be associated with considerable harm. Often probabilities of diseases or syndromes are not known, and the physician must use judgment to assign them. However, an alternative method for determining the optimal treatment is by maximizing the number of patients expected to be cured. For the same treatment values given above let F be the fraction of patients receiving T1 and (1-F) the fraction receiving T2. If all patients had disease D1, we would expect to cure $80/100 \times F + 20/100 \times (1-F)$ which equals 0.2 + 0.6 F. Similarly, if all patients had disease D2 then we would expect to cure $30/100 \times F + 90/100 (1-F)$ which equals 0.9 to 0.6 F. From these 2 equations, the number of people cured is maximized when $F = 7/12$ whereby we would expect a cure in 55% of patients. Thus, a proportion equal to 7/12 should receive treatment T1 and 5/12 should receive treatment T2. In recent years, these concepts have gained traction in the medical literature; one study demonstrated a reduction in antibiotic misuse by discretizing clinical information using a game-theoretic approach.[18] Although many other nuances may be considered in the final decisions regarding disease processes and therapies, these concepts provide a valuable workable framework to think about complex problems.

NOISE

There are two components to errors in judgment—bias and noise. Although much attention has been paid to bias, the role of noise which may be equally or more important is often ignored. To fully understand error, it is imperative, we understand both bias and noise and their relative contributions. Simply defined noise is variability in judgements that should be identical.[19] This variability may occur when different individuals judge the same situation or when the same individual judges identical situations. The simplest example of noise in medicine is 2 physicians arriving at separate the diagnosis for the same patient. Diagnosis involves judgment and obviously, the judgment of one or both physicians is incorrect (we may not know which); the divergent opinions constitute noise. It is also well known that physicians arrive at different diagnoses when presented twice with the same case.[20–22] Noise invades both diagnostic judgments as well as treatments.[23–25] On closer examination, the pervasiveness and magnitude of this phenomenon is astonishing.[26–28] Variability in judgments by the same person may be triggered by mood, fatigue, weather, and sequence effects. Perhaps the most pertinent to critical care medicine especially amid the COVID-19 pandemic are stress and fatigue. One study of over 700,000 primary care visits demonstrated that physicians were significantly more likely to prescribe opioids at the end of a long day.[29] Such patterns were not seen in prescriptions of nonsteroidal antiinflammatory drugs or physical therapy referrals.[30] Similarly, prescriptions for antibiotics were more likely while those of flu shots and cancer screenings less likely at the end of a long day.[31–33] Even more surprisingly, doctors seem to wash their hands less at the end of the day.[34] Since bias and noise play the same role in the calculation of overall error (mean squared error or MSE = bias^2 + noise^2),[19] it is quite likely that there is a hidden epidemic of undiscovered noise in the ICU. Some important examples of noise in the context of critical care include poor interobserver reliability in the interpretation of chest radiographs for the diagnosis of ARDS (reliability does not improve with training),[35] clinical assessment of work of breathing, discerning the etiology of acute kidney injury[36,37] as well as the identification and timely diagnosis of sepsis.[38] One can easily extrapolate how variability in the diagnosis of such common disorders would, in turn, lead to variability in the delivery of time-sensitive treatments such as antibiotics, volume resuscitation, and provision of appropriate techniques of mechanical ventilation. Compounding the problem and aggravating the variability in the decision-making process is the occurrence of occasion noise as a result of stress, fatigue, and mood so prevalent in high-strung ICU environments. Noise can be reduced by improvement in the skill levels of physicians[39]; appropriate training is key to the reduction of error and to the mitigation of both noise and bias. Algorithmic approaches such as deep learning and artificial intelligence are known to reduce noise.[40–42] With rapidly advancing technology, these approaches are likely to undergo refinements and become increasingly ubiquitous in the future. Until these advances can occur, a relatively simple method of reducing noise is through the implementation of guidelines. Guidelines help distill complex decisions into relatively simpler sub-decisions; judgment is not altogether eliminated but is simplified using rules and relevant predictors. Relevant examples include the ABCDEF bundle and the protocols for the early identification and treatment of sepsis, both of which have been associated with improved outcomes.[43,44]

SUMMARY

Clinical reasoning involves predictive judgment which is afflicted by systematic error which comprises bias and noise. Reasoning foundations can be mathematically described by logic, probability, and value theory. Intuitive judgment of these mathematical concepts leads to systematic errors in reasoning. Clinicians should familiarize themselves with biases and their mathematical underpinnings to improve reasoning. Noise is pervasive in medicine and may be reduced using algorithmic approaches and guidelines.

CLINICS CARE POINTS

- Clinical reasoning is afflicted by systematic errors in judgment or biases
- Misconceptions of statistical and probability concepts underpin most biases
- Intensivists should familiarize themselves with mathematical concepts to improve decision hygiene

- An equally important component to errors in judgment is noise
- Noise is pervasive and attempts should be made to reduce it

DISCLOSURE

The authors (M. Barash and R.S. Nanchal) have nothing to disclose.

REFERENCES

1. Tversky A, Kahneman D. Judgment under uncertainty: heuristics and biases. Science 1974;185(4157):1124–31.
2. Ledley RS, Lusted LB. Reasoning foundations of medical diagnosis; symbolic logic, probability, and value theory aid our understanding of how physicians reason. Science 1959;130(3366):9–21.
3. Wainer H. The most dangerous equation. Am Sci 2007;95(3):249.
4. Galton F. Natural inheritance. London: Macmillan; 1889.
5. Bar-Hillel M. On the subjective probability of compound events. Organizational Behavior & Human Performance 1973;9(3):396–406.
6. Cohen J, Chesnick EI, Haran D. Evaluation of compound probabilities in sequential choice. Nature 1971;232(5310):414–6.
7. Cahan A. Diagnosis is driven by probabilistic reasoning: counter-point. Diagnosis (Berl) 2016;3(3):99–101.
8. Bayes T, Noon J. An introduction to the doctrine of fluxions; and, Defense of the mathematicians against the objections of the author of the analyst, so far as they are designed to affect their general methods of reasoning. London: Printed for J. Noon; 1736.
9. Kline JA, Mitchell AM, Kabrhel C, et al. Clinical criteria to prevent unnecessary diagnostic testing in emergency department patients with suspected pulmonary embolism. J Thromb Haemost 2004;2(8):1247–55.
10. Wong CH, Khin LW, Heng KS, et al. The LRINEC (Laboratory Risk Indicator for Necrotizing Fasciitis) score: a tool for distinguishing necrotizing fasciitis from other soft tissue infections. Crit Care Med 2004;32(7):1535–41.
11. Bendapudi PK, Upadhyay V, Sun L, et al. Clinical scoring systems in thrombotic microangiopathies. Semin Thromb Hemost 2017;43(5):540–8.
12. Kline JA, Stubblefield WB. Clinician gestalt estimate of pretest probability for acute coronary syndrome and pulmonary embolism in patients with chest pain and dyspnea. Ann Emerg Med 2014;63(3):275–80.
13. Penaloza A, Verschuren F, Meyer G, et al. Comparison of the unstructured clinician gestalt, the wells score, and the revised Geneva score to estimate pretest probability for suspected pulmonary embolism. Ann Emerg Med 2013;62(2):117–24.e2.
14. Jain BP. Why is diagnosis not probabilistic in clinical-pathological conference (CPCs): point. Diagnosis (Berl) 2016;3(3):95–7.
15. Masi AT, Hunder GG, Lie JT, et al. The American College of Rheumatology 1990 criteria for the classification of Churg-Strauss syndrome (allergic granulomatosis and angiitis). Arthritis Rheum 1990;33(8):1094–100.
16. Pauker SG, Kassirer JP. The threshold approach to clinical decision making. N Engl J Med 1980;302(20):1109–17.
17. Neumann JV, Morgenstern O. Theory of games and economic behavior. Princeton (NJ): Princeton University Press; 1963.

18. Diamant M, Baruch S, Kassem E, et al. A game theoretic approach reveals that discretizing clinical information can reduce antibiotic misuse. Nat Commun 2021; 12(1):1148.
19. Kahneman D, Sibony O, Sunstein CR. Noise a flaw in human judgement. London: William Collins; 2021.
20. Robinson PJ, Culpan G, Wiggins M. Interpretation of selected accident and emergency radiographic examinations by radiographers: a review of 11000 cases. Br J Radiol 1999;72(858):546–51.
21. Detre KM, Wright E, Murphy ML, et al. Observer agreement in evaluating coronary angiograms. Circulation 1975;52(6):979–86.
22. Banky M, Clark RA, Pua YH, et al. Inter- and intra-rater variability of testing velocity when assessing lower limb spasticity. J Rehabil Med 2019;51(1):54–60.
23. OECD. Geographic Variations in Health Care. 2014.
24. Hurley MP, Schoemaker L, Morton JM, et al. Geographic variation in surgical outcomes and cost between the United States and Japan. Am J Manag Care 2016; 22(9):600–7.
25. Appleby J, Raleigh V, Frosini F, et al. Variations in health care: the good, the bad and the inexplicable. London: King's Fund; 2011.
26. Speciale AC, Pietrobon R, Urban CW, et al. Observer variability in assessing lumbar spinal stenosis severity on magnetic resonance imaging and its relation to cross-sectional spinal canal area. Spine (Phila Pa 1976 2002;27(10):1082–6.
27. Farmer ER, Gonin R, Hanna MP. Discordance in the histopathologic diagnosis of melanoma and melanocytic nevi between expert pathologists. Hum Pathol 1996; 27(6):528–31.
28. Palazzo JP, Hyslop T. Hyperplastic ductal and lobular lesions and carcinomas in situ of the breast: reproducibility of current diagnostic criteria among community- and academic-based pathologists. Breast J 1998;4(4):230–7.
29. Neprash HT, Barnett ML. Association of primary care clinic appointment time with opioid prescribing. JAMA Netw Open 2019;2(8):e1910373.
30. Philpot LM, Khokhar BA, Roellinger DL, et al. Time of day is associated with opioid prescribing for low back pain in primary care. J Gen Intern Med 2018; 33(11):1828–30.
31. Linder JA, Doctor JN, Friedberg MW, et al. Time of day and the decision to prescribe antibiotics. JAMA Intern Med 2014;174(12):2029–31.
32. Hsiang EY, Mehta SJ, Small DS, et al. Association of primary care clinic appointment time with clinician ordering and patient completion of breast and colorectal cancer screening. JAMA Netw Open 2019;2(5):e193403.
33. Kim RH, Day SC, Small DS, et al. Variations in influenza vaccination by clinic appointment time and an active choice intervention in the electronic health record to increase influenza vaccination. JAMA Netw Open 2018;1(5):e181770.
34. You X, Tan H, Hu S, et al. Effects of preconception counseling on maternal health care of migrant women in China: a community-based, cross-sectional survey. BMC Pregnancy Childbirth 2015;15:55.
35. Goddard SL, Rubenfeld GD, Manoharan V, et al. The randomized educational acute respiratory distress syndrome diagnosis study: a trial to improve the radiographic diagnosis of acute respiratory distress syndrome. Crit Care Med 2018; 46(5):743–8.
36. de Groot MG, de Neef M, Otten MH, et al. Interobserver Agreement on Clinical Judgment of Work of Breathing in Spontaneously Breathing Children in the Pediatric Intensive Care Unit. J Pediatr Intensive Care 2020;9(1):34–9. https://doi.org/10.1055/s-0039-1697679.

37. Koyner JL, Garg AX, Thiessen-Philbrook H, et al. Adjudication of etiology of acute kidney injury: experience from the TRIBE-AKI multi-center study. BMC Nephrol 2014;15:105.
38. Vincent JL. The clinical challenge of sepsis identification and monitoring. PLoS Med 2016;13(5):e1002022.
39. Tsugawa Y, Newhouse JP, Zaslavsky AM, et al. Physician age and outcomes in elderly patients in hospital in the US: observational study. BMJ 2017;357:j1797.
40. Rodriguez-Ruiz A, Lång K, Gubern-Merida A, et al. Stand-alone artificial intelligence for breast cancer detection in mammography: comparison with 101 radiologists. J Natl Cancer Inst 2019;111(9):916–22.
41. Richens JG, Lee CM, Johri S. Improving the accuracy of medical diagnosis with causal machine learning. Nat Commun 2020;11(1):3923.
42. Gulshan V, Peng L, Coram M, et al. Development and validation of a deep learning algorithm for detection of diabetic retinopathy in retinal fundus photographs. JAMA 2016;316(22):2402–10.
43. Seymour CW, Gesten F, Prescott HC, et al. Time to treatment and mortality during mandated emergency care for sepsis. N Engl J Med 2017;376(23):2235–44.
44. Pun BT, Balas MC, Barnes-Daly MA, et al. Caring for critically ill patients with the ABCDEF bundle: results of the ICU liberation Collaborative in over 15,000 adults. Crit Care Med 2019;47(1):3–14.

Diagnostic Stewardship
Appropriate Testing and Judicious Treatments

Yasaman Fatemi, MD[a],*, Paul A. Bergl, MD[b,c]

KEYWORDS
- Diagnostic stewardship • Diagnostic error • Overdiagnosis
- Clinical decision support • Medical-decision making

KEY POINTS
- Diagnostic stewardship is the concept of promoting timely and appropriate diagnostic testing to optimize patient outcomes and promote high-value care.
- The tenets of diagnostic stewardship include right test, right time, right patient, right interpretation, and right treatment.
- Diagnostic stewardship principles have been applied to key infectious syndromes in the ICU including bloodstream infections, urinary tract infections, ventilator-associated pneumonia, *Clostridioides difficile* colonization and infections, and central nervous system infections to optimize the diagnostic process.
- Diagnostic stewardship or safety teams, similar to antimicrobial stewardship programs, may be a potential avenue in optimizing diagnostic test utilization and interpretation in the future.
- Appropriate stewardship of diagnostic tests can help reduce false-positive test results, overdiagnosis, and health care overutilization.

INTRODUCTION

Stewardship implies a duty to responsibly manage resources. Although intensivists likely have encountered antimicrobial stewardship programs in their practice, they may lack familiarity with the more expansive – but admittedly waxy – concept of diagnostic stewardship. Proponents of diagnostic stewardship emphasize the intimate links between diagnostic testing and management decisions in infectious syndromes.[1] Principles of diagnostic stewardship have seeped into other realms of critical care medicine as a framework to inform how one qualifies the appropriateness of diagnostic testing and how one tailor interventions based on those results.[2,3] To fully understand how diagnostic stewardship will shape the future of critical care, we must first have a working definition that suits our practice.

[a] Division of Infectious Diseases, Children's Hospital of Philadelphia, 3401 Civic Center Boulevard, Philadelphia, PA 19104, USA; [b] Department of Critical Care, Gundersen Lutheran Medical Center, 1900 South Avenue, Mail Stop LM3-001, La Crosse, WI 54601, USA; [c] Department of Medicine, University of Wisconsin School of Medicine and Public Health, Madison, WI, USA
* Corresponding author.
E-mail address: fatemiy@chop.edu

Crit Care Clin 38 (2022) 69–87
https://doi.org/10.1016/j.ccc.2021.09.002
0749-0704/22/© 2021 Elsevier Inc. All rights reserved.

In this article, we will articulate a practical framework for diagnostic stewardship in the intensive care unit (ICU); this framework will be grounded in the antimicrobial stewardship movement from which diagnostic stewardship evolved. Next, we will discuss the design, implementation, and evidence for diagnostic stewardship programs in the management of infectious syndromes among the critically ill. Finally, after considering how stewardship principles and lessons apply to the diagnostic pathways of other noninfectious disorders encountered in the ICU, we will explore diagnostic stewardship at the frontiers of modern diagnostic testing.

WHAT IS DIAGNOSTIC STEWARDSHIP?

Concerns about appropriately using laboratory tests to diagnose and treat infectious diseases have existed since the 1970s.[4] With the relatively recent advent of rapid diagnostic tests – most often through nucleic acid amplification tests (NAATs) including polymerase chain reaction (PCR) techniques – infectious disease specialists recognized the promise of using these tests for timely tailoring of antimicrobial therapy.[5,6] In 2016, "diagnostic stewardship" came into common use, both through the peer-reviewed literature and through the World Health Organization (WHO).[7] Focused exclusively on infectious diseases, early proponents posited that timely, accurate microbiological data would enhance the safety and efficiency of patient management decisions.[1,7] In these early conceptualizations, diagnostic stewardship applied to all stages of the diagnostic process, from appropriate test selection and specimen collection methods (especially to reduce risks of contamination) through the consideration of epidemiologic context and clinical probabilities of disease in result interpretation.[1]

These first iterations of the diagnostic stewardship concept did not allay all long-standing problems in managing infectious syndromes. Most prominently, the sensitivity of molecular methods led to new questions about when to test patients and how to best interpret results, as exemplified by the conundrum of distinguishing colonization with *Clostridioides difficile* from true infectious colitis (as elaborated later in this chapter). As such, advocates of diagnostic stewardship widened their focus to guide appropriate clinical behavior and to reduce unnecessary testing and false-positive results.[8,9] Stewards could achieve the added goals of reducing overdiagnosis and overtreatment by avoiding running diagnostic tests on inappropriate specimens (eg, by not culturing sputum contaminated by oral flora), avoiding diagnostic tests in low pretest probability situations (eg, by restricting urine cultures to patients with active symptoms of urinary infection), cascading tests (eg, performing urine culture only if the urinalysis demonstrates pyuria), and/or nudging clinicians in the test ordering process through electronic order prompting.[8,9]

Though born of the specialty of infectious disease, the concept of diagnostic stewardship spans all disciplines, perhaps as best evidenced by the Choosing Wisely initiative.[10] Many professional societies have participated in Choosing Wisely and have highlighted appropriate use of laboratory testing as a key target. Recommendations relevant to the practice of critical care include avoiding urine culture in the absence of clinical symptoms attributable to urinary tract infection, deferring routine daily bloodwork in clinically stable patients, and avoiding thrombophilia testing in the context of acute venous thromboembolism.[10] Although not explicitly labeled as a stewardship campaign, such Choosing Wisely recommendations align with a core principle of diagnostic stewardship: clinical context is key.

Against this backdrop, one can idealize a clinical approach to diagnostic stewardship in the ICU. The intensivist acting as a steward would only order diagnostic testing based on a reasonable probability of disease and would request such testing only when it directly informs time-sensitive therapeutic decisions. Further, the ideal steward would consider improved patient outcomes – not just incremental changes in diagnostic confidence – as paramount. The steward would also understand the economic impact of testing not merely as a matter of health care expenditures but as a value-based proposition. In summary, diagnostic stewardship in the ICU boils down to ordering the "right test for the right patient at the right time."[11]

STEWARDSHIP OF KEY INFECTIOUS SYNDROMES IN THE ICU

In the critical care setting, there are several common clinical infectious syndromes and associated tests with evidence to guide testing strategies. Here we will review several common diagnostic tests and evidence to support appropriate utilization.

BLOODSTREAM INFECTIONS AND BLOOD CULTURES

One of the most commonly ordered tests in the hospital setting is blood cultures. Historically, indications for obtaining blood cultures in nonneutropenic patients have been broad and nonspecific. Clinical indications as common as fever or leukocytosis are drivers of blood cultures yet are not well-correlated with bacteremia. In adult patients, only 5% to 15% of blood cultures are positive[12] with up 50% falsely positive.[13–15] Notably, the false-positive rate for blood cultures is higher for those obtained from a central venous catheter (CVC) as compared with peripheral blood cultures.[16] Additionally, many blood cultures are obtained on patients who are already on antibiotics, further decreasing the true yield.[17] The downstream consequences of unnecessary blood cultures include longer hospital stays, increased testing and costs, and unnecessary antibiotics.[18]

The Infectious Disease Society of America (IDSA) guidelines for using the microbiology laboratory include guidance on blood culture technique and appropriate utilization. The IDSA emphasizes a preference for peripheral venipuncture method for obtaining blood cultures as this approach has decreased risk for contamination than samples obtained from CVCs.[16] Additionally, the guidelines include organism-specific recommendations including increased risk of contaminants with cultures obtained from CVCs.[16]

The yield of blood cultures can also vary based on infectious disease syndrome. One approach to guiding appropriate use of cultures has been to list low-risk scenarios for bacteremia; in these situations, routine blood cultures should not be obtained unless there is a concern for severe sepsis or septic shock. One particular proposed algorithm lists low-risk (<10% risk) scenarios including isolated fever or leukocytosis, uncomplicated cellulitis, uncomplicated cystitis, nonsevere community-acquired or hospital-acquired pneumonia, and postoperative fever within 48 hours of surgery based on the review of previous studies.[19] Although intensivists may infrequently find themselves managing lower risk patients, they should recognize that these risk-based stratifications create potential opportunities for improved clinical decision support and diagnostic stewardship of blood cultures.

Several studies have evaluated quality improvement interventions to reduce the frequency of blood cultures in multiple settings. One time-series analysis studying a quality improvement initiative at a large tertiary care children's hospital demonstrated decreased the frequency of blood cultures obtained and a decrease in CVC-derived blood cultures in a pediatric ICU.[20] This initiative involved both a fever and sepsis checklist as well as a blood culture decision algorithm. A time-series analysis of the intervention demonstrated a 46% reduction in the overall blood culture collection rate. Implementation of another clinical decision algorithm for adult patients based on risk stratification previously derived through a scoping review.[19] demonstrated a decrease in blood culture collection rate from both medical ICUs and medical units as compared with controls (which were surgical ICU and surgical floor units, respectively) without major differences in clinical outcomes or adherence to Medicare-mandated sepsis care.[21]

Blood cultures remain an important and simple diagnostic tool; however, there is increased recognition that many more blood cultures are obtained than necessary with potential downstream consequences of additional testing, prolonging hospital stay, and increasing costs. Harnessing clinical decision support, such as through risk-stratification and point-of-care guidance on best practices for collecting blood cultures, will restrict blood cultures to situations when they are necessary. In turn, such cultures should yield more valuable information and fewer false positives.

URINARY TRACT INFECTION TESTING

The diagnosis of urinary tract infections has generally been accepted in nonneutropenic patients to include signs of inflammation (ie, pyuria) and microbiologic growth on urine culture. Asymptomatic bacteriuria and sterile pyuria have been key areas of antimicrobial stewardship efforts.[22,23] Similarly, diagnostic stewardship involves the appropriate interpretation of these tests (ie, differentiating urinary tract infection from asymptomatic bacteriuria or sterile pyuria) and extends to the consideration of whether the initial ordering of the urine studies (urinalysis, urine culture) are appropriate. The initial decision to evaluate for a urinary tract infection relies on assessing the pretest probability of the patient having a urinary tract infection and considering special situations that may involve higher rates of asymptomatic bacteriuria (such as patients with indwelling urinary catheters). Here we will discuss both catheter and non–catheter-related urinary tract infection evaluation in nonneutropenic patients.

In general, ordering urinalysis and urine culture should be avoided in the absence of the associated patient symptoms.[24] This practice is particularly important in the setting of indwelling catheters, whereby pyuria can exist without true infection and whereby urine cultures on catheters may reflect rapid biofilm formation (even within hours) on the device itself rather than the evidence of infection.[24] Catheter-associated urinary tract infections account for a significant portion of antimicrobial use as well as a source of potential true infection. Urinary tract infections are one of the most common healthcare-associated infections with 70% to 80% of these occurring in the setting of indwelling urinary catheters.[25,26] Diagnostic investigation in the setting of indwelling urinary catheters relies on correlating clinical symptoms with microbiologic testing. Testing in the absence of clinical symptoms can lead to excess testing and antimicrobial use due to the inevitable presence of bacterial biofilm formation.[16,24,25]

In pediatrics, there is a similar focus on clinician risk stratification to guide initial testing for potential urinary tract infection and advise against testing in the absence of relevant clinical signs or symptoms.[27] Additionally, a two-step method of obtaining a urinalysis and only sending the sample to urine culture if there is pyuria has been shown to effectively reduce diagnosing and thus using antimicrobials for asymptomatic bacteriuria.[28]

Several diagnostic stewardship initiatives have focused on reducing the treatment of asymptomatic bacteriuria by focusing on improving appropriate testing scenarios. One such study, implemented a 2-phase stewardship program for urinary culture ordering and reporting.[29] In the first phase, the ordering clinician was required to select a patient population group and urinalysis and cultures were performed on all requested specimens; however, culture results from specimens were withheld if urinalysis did not demonstrate pyuria unless the specimen was from prespecified special population groups (transplant, oncology, pregnancy, and pediatrics) or certain sources (ureteric, suprapubic, nephrostomy tube). In the second phase, urine culture was not performed for samples that did not meet prespecified criteria or show pyuria.[29] By withholding test results, the researchers were able to demonstrate a significant decrease in antimicrobial prescribing without increasing subsequent risk of bacteremia or other adverse outcomes such as mortality.[29] Other quasi-experimental studies have affirmed that restricting urine culture to patients with pyuria does not result in a significant increase in gram-negative bacteremia.[30] Other studies have focused on single modality interventions such as education, audit and feedback, or clinical decision support. A review of implementation strategies demonstrated that multiple modalities including education, audit and feedback, clinical decision support, and bundling several types of strategies were all effective in reducing antibiotic treatment of asymptomatic bacteriuria in adult patients.[23]

TRACHEAL CULTURES AND VENTILATOR-ASSOCIATED PNEUMONIA

Ventilator-associated pneumonia (VAP) remains a pervasive diagnostic and therapeutic conundrum in the ICU. Although VAP is associated with increased morbidity and mortality,[31,32] clinicians must counterbalance against downstream effects from over-diagnosis and overtreatment, which are arguably equally pervasive.[33] However, implementing these concepts into practice still faces several hurdles.

Respiratory cultures on endotracheal secretions are commonly performed in the diagnosis of hospital-acquired or VAP. Although such cultures are part of the preferred diagnostic pathway in VAP,[34] distinguishing contamination or colonization from true pathogens may prove difficult. Further, although lower respiratory tract sampling through bronchoalveolar lavage and/or performing quantitative cultures should theoretically alleviate some of this confusion, studies have consistently failed to identify a therapeutic advantage – such as through a reduction in antibiotics or improved patient outcomes – from these diagnostic approaches.[35] Incorporating better estimates of pretest probability of VAP would enhance the utility of endotracheal aspirate cultures in suspected VAP. Clinical scoring systems, such as the Clinical Pulmonary Infection Score, unfortunately, have been plagued by poor test performance characteristics.[36]

Given these limitations and unresolved uncertainties with traditional respiratory cultures, alternative strategies are acutely needed. Targeted testing for resistant pathogens may represent one such opportunity in improving diagnostic stewardship in VAP. For example, nasal swab testing for methicillin-resistant *Staphylococcus aureus* (MRSA) using PCR has outstanding sensitivity in both community-acquired pneumonia and VAP.[37] Integrating reflexive MRSA testing on endotracheal aspirates has the potential to reduce unnecessary use of MRSA-directed antibiotics. Whether expanded microarray testing for genetic resistance markers would reduce broad-spectrum antibiotic use remains unknown.

Biomarker-informed stewardship represents another promising frontier, but studies thus far have yielded disappointing results. A recent multicenter randomized controlled trial prospectively evaluated the utility of using validated clinical biomarkers, name IL-1B and IL8, to improve antimicrobial stewardship in VAP.[38] This well-designed study embodied several aspects of diagnostic stewardship including prompt results and actionable result reporting with a clear intention of reducing unnecessary antibiotic treatment. In this trial, all patients were ventilated adults in the ICU who underwent bronchoalveolar lavage (as part of the protocol) for suspected VAP.

In the intervention arm, clinicians were provided timely guidance with an interpretative summary when IL-1B and IL-8 were below cutoffs. Specifically, clinicians were informed that "biomarker results [were] below cutoff. The negative predictive value is 1. VAP is very unlikely. Consider discontinuation of antibiotics." Despite this guidance, investigators found no difference in antibiotic-free days or any other clinically important outcome between the intervention and control arm.

Other common biomarkers like procalcitonin have an uncertain role in diagnostic stewardship for VAP. A recent meta-analysis evaluating procalcitonin's diagnostic accuracy, prognostic ability, and therapeutic efficacy in VAP identified 18 studies with a total of 1774 patients; most studies were limited to retrospective analyses or had major methodologic limitations.[39] A small reduction in the duration of antibiotics was the only relatively certain and consistent result. Although diagnostic stewardship seeks to reduce the duration of unnecessary antibiotic therapy, this outcome alone may not justify procalcitonin guidance as part of a larger VAP stewardship campaign.

Bedside clinicians tend toward caution in ventilated ICU patients even though they frequently admit to overdiagnosing and overtreating suspected VAP.[40] Frequent culturing, often in the absence of new clinical or radiographic changes, and misinterpretation of culture results tend to drive this overdiagnosis.[40] These cultural aspects of clinical care likely explain findings of "failed" stewardship trials, such as the aforementioned biomarker-based randomized control trial.[38]

Future diagnostic stewardship efforts in VAP will accordingly need to overcome challenges in diagnosis and clinicians' comfort in withholding antibiotics. A stewardship-oriented approach could integrate some assessment of both pretest probability and risk of a delayed diagnosis of VAP before allowing respiratory cultures to be ordered for patients on prolonged mechanical ventilation.[41] When obtained, culture result reporting could be also enhanced. For example, specifying that no resistant pathogens were recovered might be more encouraging to clinicians as compared with simply reporting "mixed flora present." Quantitative cultures could also be prohibited for endotracheal samples. Quantification may bias the clinician as high burdens may be perceived as more dangerous when such a burden may simply represent extensive colonization of the endotracheal tube or upper airway.

CLOSTRIDIOIDES DIFFICILE (FORMERLY CLOSTRIDIUM DIFFICILE) COLONIZATION AND INFECTION

C. difficile colitis is a relatively common hospital-associated infection and is a known consequence of broad-spectrum antimicrobial use. Antimicrobial stewardship programs often include the reduction of C. difficile colitis as an outcome of interventions given the strong link with antimicrobial use. However, C. difficile testing proves to be complex as culture is difficult and resource-intensive. Thus, like many infectious diseases, positive testing may not necessarily reflect true infection.

Diagnosis of C. difficile relies on positive test results in the appropriate clinical scenario. Without appropriate clinical symptoms and in certain ages, positive results are more likely to represent colonization and could lead to misdiagnosis. Optimal strategies for C. difficile testing have been difficult to determine. Traditionally used NAATs are very sensitive in detecting genes responsible for toxin production. However, these methods have a positive predictive value of less than 50% when the prevalence of C. difficile is low; expectedly, the positive predictive value rises with increased prevalence.[42] More recently, glutamate dehydrogenase (GDH) assays are used to detect actively growing C. difficile cells. GDH is produced by both toxigenic and nontoxigenic strains of C. difficile, but is only produced by living cells. These tests have similar sensitivity to NAATs but continue to suffer from the lack of specificity for true *C. difficile* infection. To improve the positive predictive value of *C. difficile* testing, the Infectious Diseases Society of America (IDSA) recommends either using a multistep testing algorithm that begins with either NAAT or GDH and pairs this with confirmation of toxin enzyme immunoassay. Alternatively, NAAT can be used alone if an institution uses prespecified specimen submission guidance. This prespecified guidance reflects testing in the appropriate clinical setting. The IDSA recommends focusing testing efforts on those patients with new-onset and unexplained symptoms of 3 or more loose stools in 24 hours. Additionally, to increase the likelihood that the symptoms could be explained by *C. difficile*, patients with recent laxative use or stools that are not truly loose should be excluded from testing.[42]

The importance of appropriate patient testing is particularly apparent in the pediatric patient population. There is a high rate of asymptomatic *C. difficile* colonization in infants and young children, particularly those under 2 years of age. Most infants are colonized with nontoxigenic strains; however, colonization with toxigenic strains also occurs, yet does not necessarily cause symptoms. In infants, colonization rates can exceed 40%, so testing of children under 2 years of age is discouraged and should only be considered in select cases.[42]

Diagnostic stewardship of *C. difficile* testing has been focused on both testing the right patient and right time as well as using the correct test to improve interpretation.[42,43] As the advent of more sensitive molecular techniques for *C. difficile* detection, there has been increasing concern about the overdiagnosis of *C. difficile* infections.[43]

Stewardship and quality improvement initiatives have focused on electronic ordering guidance, testing algorithms, and clinician education to help exclude these specimens. In pediatrics, strategies have focused on excluding testing of patients under 1 year of age and limiting testing under 2 years of age.[42,44,45] In adult patients, both testing algorithms and embedded order guidance have been used, both of which have been shown to decrease inappropriate testing.[42,46–48] In addition to interventions targeting the ordering phase, there are diagnostic stewardship initiatives for both pediatric and adult patients at the laboratory level whereby specimens that do not meet certain criteria – such as those collected more than 24 hours after the initial order, tests on the formed stool, or tests for patients on laxatives at the time of collection – are canceled or refused.[45,47,49] Interventions at both the ordering and laboratory phases have been effective, demonstrating an area ripe for collaboration between clinical and laboratory medicine colleagues. The outcomes of these initiatives primarily focus on decreased antimicrobial utilization and decreased cost. Further work is needed to better define *C. difficile* infection from colonization to truly distinguish appropriate testing contexts.

CENTRAL NERVOUS SYSTEM INFECTIONS

Intensivists often evaluate patients with suspected central nervous system (CNS) infection. Unfortunately, an underdeveloped and conflicting evidence base[50–53] and lack of guidelines may leave the diagnostic steward with little choice but to err on the side of performing lumbar puncture (LP) in critically ill patients with a modest pretest probability for CNS infection. Among immunocompetent critically ill surgical patients who have not suffered head trauma or undergone neurosurgical intervention, the yield of LP is likely exceedingly low.[52] Further, nosocomial CNS infection is rare,[50,51] and LP can likely be deferred for this indication. However, clinical parameters alone are not reliably associated with the likelihood of an abnormal cerebrospinal fluid (CSF) profile.[54] Prospective studies evaluating objective criteria for performing LP among ICU patients are sorely needed to inform stewardship algorithms.

Once LP has been performed, the question of appropriate PCR microarray testing for pathogens causing meningitis or encephalitis also remains unsettled. In one retrospective single-center cohort study, restricting such testing to patients with CSF pleocytosis in a diagnostic stewardship model proved largely safe and seems to have improved the yield of the microarray panel.[55] Among the 459 microarray tests ordered, 196 (43%) were rejected due to a lack of pleocytosis. Subsequent diagnostic testing with more traditional microbiological methods ultimately identified only 4 cases of CNS infection among these 196 rejected samples; all 4 infections involved herpesviruses and occurred in immunocompromised hosts who presumably lacked effective immune responses. As such, this study supports the practice of restricting microarray PCR testing to immunocompetent adults with CSF pleocytosis or the immunocompromised.

A separate retrospective analysis of 1025 CSF specimens in 948 distinct pediatric patients found that CSF markers of inflammation were poor predictors of positive microarray PCR testing.[56] In this children's hospital, microarray PCR testing was not restricted to patients with CSF pleocytosis. Most commonly, viral pathogens would have been missed in this cohort if microarray testing was restricted to pediatric patients with CSF pleocytosis, abnormally high CSF protein, or abnormally low CSF glucose levels. Surprisingly, 35.5% of the positive microarray PCR tests were accompanied by a completely benign CSF (ie, white blood cell counts <5 per high powered field, normal protein, and normal glucose) and most often consisted of viral pathogens for which there is no specific treatment beyond supportive care. Additionally, the negative predictive value for the absence of pleocytosis was nonetheless a robust 94.0%.

Together, these studies suggest that strictly prohibiting the use of microarray testing on patients with an abnormal CSF profile would lead to occasional missed diagnoses, mostly of viral pathogens for which there is no specific antimicrobial agent. A stewardship model for microarray PCR testing could require clinicians to review the results of the basic CSF profile (cell count, protein, and glucose) before allowing orders for the microarray panel. Such a system, however, would need to allow bedside clinicians to override clinical decision support restrictions in high pretest probability situations and among the immunocompromised.

STEWARDSHIP DURING AN INFECTIOUS PANDEMIC

Finally, the recent COVID-19 pandemic has highlighted how diagnostic stewardship may intersect with testing for emerging novel pathogens. Early in the pandemic, a stewardship-oriented mindset was required for allocating testing resources, particularly when testing was highly limited and when test performance characteristics of available tests were largely unknown.[57] In the stewardship framework, scarce testing resources for SARS-CoV-2 were often prioritized based on epidemiologic risk factors for exposure, risk for the adverse outcome from COVID-19, and patient acuity. As testing became widespread, other stewardship questions arose, such as around the issue of when and how to retest and how to interpret positive test results after apparent clinical recovery. On the side, some argued for repeated testing to enhance sensitivity in symptomatic patients when false negatives were suspected.[58] On the other side, some questioned the utility of repeat testing within a short time frame after a negative result.[59] Resolving these vexing questions lies beyond our scope; however, intensivists managing patients during future pandemics must be mindful of the broader stewardship principles involved in test ordering and allocation.

BROADER LESSONS LEARNED FROM ANTIMICROBIAL STEWARDSHIP

The larger antimicrobial stewardship movement has generated other ideas for enhancing diagnostics in the ICU; these improvements have been achieved largely by embedding clinicians in designing workflows for each phase of laboratory testing.[60] Most importantly, stewardship programs have improved patient outcomes by integrating team members who are capable of both interpreting test results and using them to guide timely decisions.[60,61] Although such skills are essential to any competent clinician's repertoire, the rapid proliferation, and sophistication of modern diagnostic tests have rendered necessary an additional layer of scrutiny brought by antimicrobial stewardship teams. Preliminary work by Laposata and colleagues has substantiated the efficacy of an analogous "diagnostic management team"[62–64] that provides clinical laboratory-based consultation for bleeding and thrombosis cases. Not only do these teams identify frequent errors of misutilization of laboratory tests,[62] but their interpretations of coagulation studies improve clinicians' satisfaction, efficiency, and perceived accuracy.[64]

Diagnostic management teams need not only focus on challenging coagulation cases but could aid in laboratory test selection and interpretation in other complex cases.[65] For example, as "-omics" such as pharmacogenomics seep into personalized ICU care, intensivists may need to lean on laboratory-based consultants to translate test results into appropriate drug selection and dosing.[66] Such changes would require fundamental changes in the scope and workload of clinical laboratory physicians[67] but may pay dividends through more efficient resource utilization and better outcomes.

Stewardship programs also attend to how results are presented. Examples include withholding in vitro antimicrobial sensitivities for antibacterials with inadequate in vivo activity or explicitly reporting likely contaminants or colonizing microbes.[60,68] Although interpretive summaries and suggested management strategies have proliferated in result reporting of laboratory tests,[60,68] such improvements could also facilitate clinical management decisions based on imaging or other novel diagnostics. For instance, echocardiography reports may flummox the ordering physician, who is often a non-cardiologist unfamiliar with measured parameters.[69] An interpretation that is "clinically driven and oriented toward the disease management and treatment"[70] would refine bedside decision-making and would ensure echocardiography is ordered judiciously.

The tenets of diagnostic stewardship in critical care can be summarized in the following table (**Table 1**).

STEWARDSHIP TEAMS? OR DIAGNOSTIC SAFETY TEAMS?

Although antimicrobial stewardship programs arose from specific needs around infectious disease testing and restricting antiinfectives to appropriate scenarios, preliminary evidence suggests such teams could also reduce diagnostic errors. Investigators at a tertiary children's hospital retrospectively examined a cohort of "great catches" that were self-identified by the antimicrobial stewardship team; these great catches included team-initiated interventions that positively influenced the patient's clinical trajectory.[71] Diagnostic errors comprised 12% of the cohort of stewardship team's great catches.[71] In other words, the stewardship team corrected a meaningful number of diagnostic errors in near real-time. In a retrospective review of 500 randomly selected hospitalized patients who received a course of antimicrobial therapy at a Veterans Affairs hospital, a separate set of investigators found diagnostic errors among 31% of cases.[72] Further, even among accurately diagnosed patients, antimicrobial selection frequently was inappropriate.[72] These findings further substantiate the role of a "second set of eyes" in reviewing microbiologic data and other clinical parameters.

Table 1
Tenets of diagnostic stewardship

Tenet of Stewardship	Key Elements of Tenet	Phases of Test Processing	Examples
Right test	Diagnostic test performance Diagnostic yield Feasibility and cost	Preanalytic (ie, before the test is performed)	Computerized order entry system prohibits testing for *C. difficile* if appropriate test was performed in the last 7 d.
		Analytical (ie, during test performance)	Urine cultures are only performed if pyuria is present.
Right patient	Appropriate indications Appropriate specimen type	Preanalytic	Molecular testing for cytomegalovirus in lower respiratory tract specimens is restricted to immunocompromised patients or to infectious disease specialist recommendations. Direct immunofluorescence antibody testing for *Pneumocystis* is only acceptable on specimens obtained from bronchoalveolar lavage.
Right time	Test turnaround time	Preanalytic	Point-of-care blood gas analyzer is added to ICU whereby utilization is high and timeliness of results is critical.
		Analytical	Microarray PCR testing is tested on blood cultures from ICU to evaluate for genetic markers of antimicrobial resistance (in advance of traditional culture and susceptibility testing).
		Postanalytic (ie, after the test has resulted)	The laboratory notifies the on-call pharmacist or intensivist with positive microarray results from blood cultures as soon as available.

(continued on next page)

Tenet of Stewardship	Key Elements of Tenet	Phases of Test Processing	Examples
Table 1 *(continued)*			
Right interpretation	Selective reporting of results Clinician-oriented guidance with results	Postanalytic	Respiratory cultures growing *Candida* species are accompanied by guidance that the result likely represents airway colonization rather than true pathogen in lower respiratory tract. Urinary antigen testing for *Legionella* is accompanied by a disclaimer that only the epidemic serotype is detected by the assay.
Right treatment	Clinical support for treatment decisions	Postanalytic	Clinical pathologist or hematologist assists in blood product ordering for patients with confusing results on rotational thromboelastometry testing.

Data from Morgan DJ, Malani P, Diekema DJ. Diagnostic Stewardship-Leveraging the Laboratory to Improve Antimicrobial Use. JAMA. 2017;318(7):607-608. https://doi.org/10.1001/jama.2017.8531; and Messacar K, Parker SK, Todd JK, Dominguez SR. Implementation of Rapid Molecular Infectious Disease Diagnostics: the Role of Diagnostic and Antimicrobial Stewardship. J Clin Microbiol. 2017;55(3):715-723. https://doi.org/10.1128/JCM.02264-16.

In light of these studies, we might reimagine stewardship teams as an additional layer of diagnostic security. The stewardship's team expanded role in the diagnostic process would need to consider clinicians' fear of overinvolvement though available evidence suggests such fears may be unfounded. Typically, stewardship teams make recommendations in only a minority of cases, most often recommend antibiotic cessation, and usually provide recommendations that are accepted by treating clinicians.[73,74] Explicitly tasking stewardship teams with providing diagnostic consultation, however, still merits additional investigation.

STEWARDSHIP, OVERDIAGNOSIS, AND RELATED CONCEPTS

Diagnostic stewardship's fundamental aim is to ensure that the right tests are ordered for the right patients at the right time, but its secondary benefits include a reduction in false positives and cases of overdiagnosis and related phenomena. Under the strictest definition, overdiagnosis occurs when clinicians make diagnoses that would never have caused symptoms or harm during the patient's lifetime.[75] Classic examples include indolent cancers detected during screening tests and asymptomatic disorders like subclinical hypothyroidism that are only discovered through aggressive case-finding. However, in a broader sense overdiagnosis may refer to any situation in which a disease or disorder is identified but for which treatment has no net benefit or causes net harm.[75,76] Thus, as cancer screening bears little relevance to critical care, intensivists routinely encounter more pervasive forms of overdiagnosis and the related problems of disease mongering, over-detection, and overutilization.[76] An overview of these terms and examples germane to critical care are shown in **Table 2**.

Overdiagnosis is most likely to occur in critical care when clinicians indiscriminately apply diagnostic tests without considering base rates of disease or the potential implications of positive test results. Sending an array of exquisitely sensitive microbiological tests on bronchial washings may reveal the presence of cytomegalovirus or *Pneumocystis jirovecii* DNA in the absence of clinical infection (ie, pneumonitis or pneumonia).[77,78] Subjecting every acutely ill patient with respiratory failure to computed tomography with pulmonary angiography may simply lead to the discovery of more subsegmental pulmonary emboli without affecting the morbidity or mortality from venous thromboembolism.[79] Performing point-of-care ultrasound on all ICU patients with sepsis might identify a subset of patients that develop transiently depressed left ventricular function but may have no clear therapeutic or prognostic implications.[80] In these examples, the harms of overdiagnosis become clear as discovering false positives may lead to unnecessary and potentially harmful treatments such as antivirals, anticoagulation, or neurohormonal blockade.

Although over-detection and overutilization are conceptually similar to overdiagnosis (see **Table 2**), the concept of disease mongering merits its own discussion. This

Table 2
Definitions and examples of overdiagnosis and related concepts

Term	Definition	Potential Examples in Critical Care
Overdiagnosis	Identification of diseases or conditions that could have remained undiscovered without causing symptoms or adversely affecting patient outcomes	Subsegmental pulmonary emboli discovered during computed tomography of the chest Incidental diagnosis of depressed left ventricular systolic function by point-of-care ultrasound in a patient with no signs of inadequate cardiac output or cardiac ischemia Diagnosis of euthyroid sick syndrome in a patient without signs or symptoms attributable to acute thyrotoxicosis or severe hypothyroidism
Disease mongering	Expansion of boundaries of illness or disease definitions in ways that do not have clear therapeutic implications and may even result in net patient harm	Diagnosing and treating all patients who "screen positive" for sepsis with aggressive fluid resuscitation and broad-spectrum antibiotics
Over-detection	Identification of health concerns that may ultimately be relevant but that are not germane to managing critical illness	Incidental pulmonary nodules or adrenal adenomas were discovered on computed tomography performed for other reasons
Overutilization	Practices and tests that are considered reasonable in the provision of critical care but that do not improve diagnostic accuracy, do not have clear treatment implications, or do not affect patient outcomes	Trending cardiac-specific troponins for a patient in whom there is a low suspicion of acute plaque rupture or for whom invasive coronary angiography is contraindicated

concept arose from concerns that pharmaceutical companies were driving overmedicalization as expanding disease definitions led to new opportunities to market new treatments.[81] Although critical care has historically not been a prime target of the pharmaceutical industry, there are 2 major implications of disease mongering to consider nonetheless. First, earlier detection and intervention for impending critical illness remains an area of intense study. Tools such as artificial intelligence-enabled risk prediction scores may avert clinical deterioration in some patients but may also subject another set of patients to unnecessarily aggressive monitoring or treatment. Second, definitions of critical illness syndromes like sepsis and acute respiratory distress syndrome (ARDS) are perpetually evolving. To avoid the harms of disease mongering, these definitions must continually seek to optimize the balance of sensitivity and specificity rather than seeking to enhance case-finding alone. Further, campaigns to promote greater awareness of conditions like sepsis must also recognize the risks of over-detection and over-labeling.

Because overdiagnosis and related problems are not isolated to unscrupulous or overzealous clinicians, solutions to overdiagnosis must address the underlying, intersecting causes. Deviations from an idealized diagnostic pathway usually arise from the complex interaction of individual, interpersonal, environmental, and organizational factors.[82–84] On the individual level, patients and clinicians are susceptible to cognitive biases that affect medical decisions[85]; most notably, clinicians tend to overestimate benefits and underestimate harms in both diagnostic testing and treatment decisions.[86] Further, the culture of health care tends to prioritize diagnostic certainty, which, in the context of proliferating and easily accessible diagnostic technology, drives overuse.[82] Given the life-threatening nature of the critical illness, intensivists may feel especially pressured to enhance clinical certainty. Deep organizational and cultural changes will likely be needed to stem the tide of overdiagnosis.

DIAGNOSTIC STEWARDSHIP ON THE FRONTIER OF CRITICAL CARE

The critical care community has witnessed a recent explosion of interest in subphenotypes of clinical syndromes.[87] Subphenotyping may transform the contemporary practice of critical care by elucidating new mechanisms of disease, enriching clinical studies, and personalizing care for our patients.[87] However, the growth of subphenotyping will undoubtedly intersect with broader dialogues around diagnostic stewardship in the ICU.

Because common critical illness syndromes, such as ARDS and sepsis, encompass a broad array of clinically heterogenous phenotypes, researchers, and clinicians alike would benefit from parsing these syndromes into subtypes. Indeed, practicing intensivists have long recognized the necessity of identifying "subphenotypes" of ARDS[88]; these have included differentiating ARDS based on mechanism of syndrome initiation, for example, direct lung injury from chemical pneumonitis versus indirect injury from extrapulmonary systemic inflammatory response, or differential responses to treatment such positive end-expiratory pressure.[87,88] Modern subphenotyping involves specifying unique diagnostic profiles of these syndromes, such as through patterns of biomarker elaboration or genetic signatures.

How should one use the lens of diagnostic stewardship to critically appraise the future of subphenotyping? Above all, the steward would demand that expanded diagnostic testing of critically ill patients would translate to tangible improvements in patient outcomes. As a precise diagnostic tool, subphenotyping could resolve management questions, such as how to optimally define critical illness-related adrenal insufficiency.[89] If subphenotyping septic shock constrained the use of stress dose steroids to patients who experienced improved outcomes with these agents, then genomic, proteomic, and biomarker signatures – ostensibly provided in a timely manner – should be incorporated into routine clinical care. Such an approach aligns with the broad tenets of diagnostic stewardship. On the contrary, introducing new diagnostic subphenotypes that lack specific therapeutic consequences may sow confusion; perhaps we should retain broad syndromic monikers like "sepsis" if enhanced diagnostic labels simply tax our cognition.

Our care delivery systems would also need refinement. First, we would need to counterbalance expanded diagnostic testing against the inconvenience to staff and harm to patients. ICU patients already are subjected to excessive phlebotomy,[90] so biomarker profiles relying on blood samples should minimize the burden of hospital-acquired anemia. Although the impact of staff workload on patient outcomes lies beyond our scope, we must recognize that gleaning marginally helpful to enhance subphenotyping may not represent appropriate resource utilization. Further, because successful diagnostic stewardship in antimicrobial management includes therapeutic guidance, we should expect laboratory reporting systems to interpret biomarker patterns or synthesize genomic and metabolomic data into clinically meaningful summaries of subphenotypes. Such summaries would, in turn, inform the bedside clinician's therapeutic decision-making.

CLINICS CARE POINTS

- Appropriate use of bacterial cultures in the ICU requires a high pretest probability and proper specimen selection. Blood cultures should be obtained peripherally, and urine cultures should only be obtained in the presence of symptoms and microscopic evidence of pyuria.
- Separating true cases of Clostridioides difficile colitis from false positives can be aided through electronic ordering guidance, testing cascades, and clinician education.
- Antibiotic stewardship teams may potentially improve diagnostic accuracy by providing a second review of clinical data.
- Bedside clinicians embody the principles of stewardship if they only pursue diagnostic testing with therapeutic or prognostic implications. Further, the bedside steward will consider both the risks of missed diagnosis and the harms of over-detection, over-treatment, and overutilization.

ACKNOWLEDGMENTS

Dr Fatemi received funding from the Gordon and Betty Moore Foundation (grant number# GBMF7276) as part of the Society to Improve Diagnosis in Medicine (SIDM) Fellowship in Diagnostic Excellence.

DISCLOSURE

Y. Fatemi and P. Bergl have no disclosures or conflicts of interest

REFERENCES

1. Dik J-WH, Poelman R, Friedrich AW, et al. An integrated stewardship model: anti-microbial, infection prevention and diagnostic (AID). Future Microbiol 2016;11(1): 93–102.
2. Tchou MJ, May S, Holcomb J, et al. Reducing point-of-care blood gas testing in the intensive care unit through diagnostic stewardship: a value improvement project. Pediatr Qual Saf 2020;5(4):e284.

3. Shokoohi H, Duggan NM, Adhikari S, et al. Point-of-care ultrasound stewardship. J Am Coll Emerg Physicians Open 2020;1(6):1326–31.

4. Bartlett RC. Medical microbiology: quality cost and clinical relevance. Wiley; 1974.

5. Goff DA, Jankowski C, Tenover FC. Using rapid diagnostic tests to optimize antimicrobial selection in antimicrobial stewardship programs. Pharmacotherapy 2012;32(8):677–87.

6. O'Brien DJ, Gould IM. Maximizing the impact of antimicrobial stewardship: the role of diagnostics, national and international efforts. Curr Opin Infect Dis 2013; 26(4):352–8.

7. Global Antimicrobial Resistance Surveillance System (GLASS). In: Diagnostic stewardship: a guide to implementation in antimicrobial resistance surveillance sites. World Health Organization. Geneva (Switzerland): World Health organization; 2016. p. 27.

8. Morgan DJ, Malani P, Diekema DJ. Diagnostic stewardship-leveraging the laboratory to improve antimicrobial Use. JAMA 2017;318(7):607–8.

9. Dyar OJ, Moran-Gilad J, Greub G, et al. ESGMD executive committee and the ESGAP executive committee. Diagnostic stewardship: are we using the right term? Clin Microbiol Infect 2019;25(3):272–3.

10. Baird GS. The choosing wisely initiative and laboratory test stewardship. Diagnosis (Berl) 2019;6(1):15–23.

11. Messacar K, Parker SK, Todd JK, et al. Implementation of rapid molecular infectious disease diagnostics: the role of diagnostic and antimicrobial stewardship. J Clin Microbiol 2017;55(3):715–23.

12. Bates DW, Cook EF, Goldman L, et al. Predicting bacteremia in hospitalized patients. A prospectively validated model. Ann Intern Med 1990;113(7):495–500.

13. Bates DW, Goldman L, Lee TH. Contaminant blood cultures and resource utilization. The true consequences of false-positive results. JAMA 1991;265(3):365–9.

14. Shafazand S, Weinacker AB. Blood cultures in the critical care unit: improving utilization and yield. Chest 2002;122(5):1727–36.

15. Lamy B, Dargère S, Arendrup MC, et al. How to optimize the use of blood cultures for the diagnosis of bloodstream infections? A State-of-the Art. Front Microbiol 2016;7. https://doi.org/10.3389/fmicb.2016.00697.

16. Miller JM, Binnicker MJ, Campbell S, et al. A guide to utilization of the microbiology laboratory for diagnosis of infectious diseases: 2018 update by the infectious diseases society of America and the American society for microbiology. Clin Infect Dis 2018;67(6):e1–94.

17. Grace CJ, Lieberman J, Pierce K, et al. Usefulness of blood culture for hospitalized patients who are receiving antibiotic therapy. Clin Infect Dis 2001;32(11):1651–5.

18. Alahmadi YM, Aldeyab MA, McElnay JC, et al. Clinical and economic impact of contaminated blood cultures within the hospital setting. J Hosp Infect 2011; 77(3):233–6.

19. Fabre V, Sharara SL, Salinas AB, et al. Does this patient need blood cultures? A scoping review of indications for blood cultures in adult Nonneutropenic Inpatients. Clin Infect Dis 2020;71(5):1339–47.

20. Woods-Hill CZ, Fackler J, Nelson McMillan K, et al. Association of a clinical practice guideline with blood culture use in critically ill children. JAMA Pediatr 2017; 171(2):157–64.

21. Fabre V, Klein E, Salinas AB, et al. A diagnostic stewardship intervention to improve blood culture use among adult Nonneutropenic Inpatients: the DISTRIBUTE study. J Clin Microbiol 2020;58(10). https://doi.org/10.1128/JCM.01053-20.

22. Köves B, Cai T, Veeratterapillay R, et al. Benefits and harms of treatment of asymp-tomatic bacteriuria: a systematic review and meta-analysis by the European asso-ciation of urology urological infection guidelines panel. Eur Urol 2017;72(6):865–8.
23. Daniel M, Keller S, Mozafarihashjin M, et al. An implementation guide to reducing overtreatment of asymptomatic bacteriuria. JAMA Intern Med 2018;178(2):271–6.
24. Morgan DJ, Croft LD, Deloney V, et al. Choosing wisely in healthcare epidemiology and antimicrobial stewardship. Infect Control Hosp Epidemiol 2016;37(7):755–60.
25. Lo E, Nicolle LE, Coffin SE, et al. Strategies to prevent catheter-associated urinary tract infections in acute care hospitals: 2014 update. Infect Control Hosp Epide-miol 2014;35(5):464–79.
26. Weber DJ, Sickbert-Bennett EE, Gould CV, et al. Incidence of catheter-associated and non-catheter-associated urinary tract infections in a healthcare system. Infect Control Hosp Epidemiol 2011;32(8):822–3.
27. Infection S on UT, management SC on QI and. Urinary tract infection: clinical practice guideline for the diagnosis and management of the initial UTI in Febrile infants and children 2 to 24 Months. Pediatrics 2011;128(3):595–610.
28. Lavelle JM, Blackstone MM, Funari MK, et al. Two-step process for ED UTI screening in febrile young children: reducing catheterization rates. Pediatrics 2016;138(1). https://doi.org/10.1542/peds.2015-3023.
29. Lee ALH, Leung ECM, Lee MKP, et al. Diagnostic stewardship programme for urine culture: impact on antimicrobial prescription in a multi-centre cohort. J Hosp Infect 2021;108:81–9. https://doi.org/10.1016/j.jhin.2020.10.027.
30. Claeys KC, Zhan M, Pineles L, et al. Conditional reflex to urine culture: evaluation of a diagnostic stewardship intervention within the Veterans' Affairs and centers for disease control and prevention practice-based Research Network. Infect Con-trol Hosp Epidemiol 2021;42(2):176–81.
31. Blot S, Koulenti D, Dimopoulos G, et al. Prevalence, risk factors, and mortality for ventilator-associated pneumonia in middle-aged, old, and very old critically ill pa-tients*. Crit Care Med 2014;42(3):601–9.
32. Melsen WG, Rovers MM, Groenwold RHH, et al. Attributable mortality of ventilator-associated pneumonia: a meta-analysis of individual patient data from randomised prevention studies. Lancet Infect Dis 2013;13(8):665–71.
33. Nussenblatt V, Avdic E, Berenholtz S, et al. Ventilator-associated pneumonia: overdiagnosis and treatment are common in medical and surgical intensive care units. Infect Control Hosp Epidemiol 2014;35(3):278–84.
34. Kalil AC, Metersky ML, Klompas M, et al. Management of adults with hospital-acquired and ventilator-associated pneumonia: 2016 clinical practice guidelines by the infectious diseases society of America and the American Thoracic society. Clin Infect Dis 2016;63(5):e61–111.
35. Berton DC, Kalil AC, Teixeira PJZ. Quantitative versus qualitative cultures of res-piratory secretions for clinical outcomes in patients with ventilator-associated pneumonia. Cochrane Database Syst Rev 2014;10:CD006482. https://doi.org/10.1002/14651858.CD006482.pub4.
36. Shan J, Chen H-L, Zhu J-H. Diagnostic accuracy of clinical pulmonary infection score for ventilator-associated pneumonia: a meta-analysis. Respir Care 2011;56(8):1087–94.
37. Parente DM, Cunha CB, Mylonakis E, et al. The clinical utility of methicillin-resistant Staphylococcus aureus (MRSA) nasal screening to Rule Out MRSA pneumonia: a diagnostic meta-analysis with antimicrobial stewardship implica-tions. Clin Infect Dis 2018;67(1):1–7.

38. Hellyer TP, McAuley DF, Walsh TS, et al. Biomarker-guided antibiotic stewardship in suspected ventilator-associated pneumonia (VAPrapid2): a randomised controlled trial and process evaluation. Lancet Respir Med 2020;8(2):182–91.
39. Alessandri F, Pugliese F, Angeletti S, et al. Procalcitonin in the assessment of ventilator associated pneumonia: a systematic review. Adv Exp Med Biol 2021; 1323:103–14. https://doi.org/10.1007/5584_2020_591.
40. Kenaa B, O'Hara LM, Richert ME, et al. A qualitative assessment of the diagnosis and management of ventilator-associated pneumonia among critical care clinicians exploring opportunities for diagnostic stewardship. Infect Control Hosp Epidemiol 2021;1–7. https://doi.org/10.1017/ice.2021.130.
41. Kenaa B, Richert ME, Claeys KC, et al. Ventilator-associated pneumonia: diagnostic test stewardship and relevance of culturing practices. Curr Infect Dis Rep 2019;21(12):50.
42. McDonald LC, Gerding DN, Johnson S, et al. Clinical practice guidelines for Clostridium difficile infection in adults and children: 2017 update by the infectious diseases society of America (IDSA) and society for healthcare epidemiology of America (SHEA). Clin Infect Dis 2018;66(7):e1–48.
43. Polage CR, Gyorke CE, Kennedy MA, et al. Overdiagnosis of Clostridium difficile infection in the molecular test Era. JAMA Intern Med 2015;175(11):1792–801.
44. Nicholson MR, Freswick PN, Di Pentima MC, et al. The use of a computerized provider order entry alert to decrease rates of Clostridium difficile testing in young pediatric patients. Infect Control Hosp Epidemiol 2017;38(5):542–6.
45. Klatte JM, Selvarangan R, Jackson MA, et al. Reducing overutilization of testing for Clostridium difficile infection in a pediatric hospital system: a quality improvement initiative. Hosp Pediatr 2016;6(1):9–14.
46. White DR, Hamilton KW, Pegues DA, et al. The impact of a computerized clinical decision support tool on inappropriate Clostridium difficile testing. Infect Control Hosp Epidemiol 2017;38(10):1204–8.
47. Madden GR, Weinstein RA, Sifri CD. Diagnostic stewardship for healthcare-associated infections: opportunities and challenges to safely reduce test Use. Infect Control Hosp Epidemiol 2018;39(2):214–8.
48. Thompson I, Lavelle C, Leonard L. An evaluation of the effectiveness of an algorithm intervention in reducing inappropriate faecal samples sent for Clostridium difficile testing. J Infect Prev 2016;17(6):278–86.
49. Truong CY, Gombar S, Wilson R, et al. Real-time electronic tracking of diarrheal episodes and laxative therapy enables verification of Clostridium difficile clinical testing criteria and reduction of Clostridium difficile infection rates. J Clin Microbiol 2017;55(5):1276–84.
50. Metersky ML, Williams A, Rafanan AL. Retrospective analysis: are fever and altered mental status indications for lumbar puncture in a hospitalized patient who has not undergone neurosurgery? Clin Infect Dis 1997;25(2):285–8.
51. Jackson WL, Shorr AF. The yield of lumbar puncture to exclude nosocomial meningitis as aetiology for mental status changes in the medical intensive care unit. Anaesth Intensive Care 2006;34(1):21–4.
52. Adelson-Mitty J, Fink MP, Lisbon A. The value of lumbar puncture in the evaluation of critically ill, non-immunosuppressed, surgical patients: a retrospective analysis of 70 cases. Intensive Care Med 1997;23(7):749–52.
53. Khasawneh FA, Smalligan RD, Mohamad TN, et al. Lumbar puncture for suspected meningitis after intensive care unit admission is likely to change management. Hosp Pract (1995) 2011;39(1):141–5.

54. Nothem M, Salazar A, Nanchal R, et al. 761: diagnostic yield of lumbar puncture in critically ill medical patients with altered mental status. Crit Care Med 2021; 49(1). Avaialble at: https://journals.lww.com/ccmjournal/Fulltext/2021/01001/761__Diagnostic_Yield_of_Lumbar_Puncture_in.729.aspx.

55. Broadhurst MJ, Dujari S, Budvytiene I, et al. Utilization, yield, and accuracy of the FilmArray meningitis/encephalitis panel with diagnostic stewardship and testing algorithm. J Clin Microbiol 2020;58(9):e00311-20.

56. Precit MR, Yee R, Pandey U, et al. Cerebrospinal fluid findings are poor predictors of appropriate FilmArray meningitis/encephalitis panel utilization in pediatric patients. J Clin Microbiol 2020;58(3):e01592-015919.

57. Shah AS, Tande AJ, Challener DW, et al. Diagnostic stewardship: an essential Element in a rapidly evolving COVID-19 pandemic. Mayo Clin Proc 2020; 95(9S):S17-9.

58. Ramdas K, Darzi A, Jain S. "Test, re-test, re-test": using inaccurate tests to greatly increase the accuracy of COVID-19 testing. Nat Med 2020;26(6):810-1.

59. Greene DN, Dickerson JA, Greninger AL, et al. When to retest: an examination of repeat COVID-19 PCR patterns in an Ambulatory population. J Clin Microbiol 2020;58(9):e01179-011720.

60. Patel R, Fang FC. Diagnostic stewardship: opportunity for a laboratory-infectious diseases partnership. Clin Infect Dis 2018;67(5):799-801.

61. Banerjee R, Teng CB, Cunningham SA, et al. Randomized trial of rapid multiplex polymerase chain reaction-based blood culture identification and susceptibility testing. Clin Infect Dis 2015;61(7):1071-80.

62. Sarkar MK, Botz CM, Laposata M. An assessment of overutilization and underutilization of laboratory tests by expert physicians in the evaluation of patients for bleeding and thrombotic disorders in clinical context and in real time. Diagnosis (Berl) 2017;4(1):21-6.

63. Marques MB, Anastasi J, Ashwood E, et al. The clinical pathologist as consultant. Am J Clin Pathol 2011;135(1):11-2.

64. Laposata ME, Laposata M, Van Cott EM, et al. Physician survey of a laboratory medicine interpretive service and evaluation of the influence of interpretations on laboratory test ordering. Arch Pathol Lab Med 2004;128(12):1424-7.

65. Verna R, Velazquez AB, Laposata M. Reducing diagnostic errors Worldwide through diagnostic management teams. Ann Lab Med 2019;39(2):121-4.

66. Peterson JF, Field JR, Shi Y, et al. Attitudes of clinicians following large-scale pharmacogenomics implementation. Pharmacogenomics J 2016;16(4):393-8.

67. Laposata M. Putting the patient first–using the expertise of laboratory professionals to produce rapid and accurate diagnoses. Lab Med 2014;45(1):4-5.

68. Dighe AS, Soderberg BL, Laposata M. Narrative interpretations for clinical laboratory evaluations: an overview. Am J Clin Pathol 2001;116(Suppl):S123-8.

69. Bansal M, Sengupta PP. How to interpret an echocardiography report (for the non-imager)? Heart 2017;103(21):1733-44.

70. Galderisi M, Cosyns B, Edvardsen T, et al. Standardization of adult transthoracic echocardiography reporting in agreement with recent chamber quantification, diastolic function, and heart valve disease recommendations: an expert consensus document of the European Association of Cardiovascular Imaging. Eur Heart J Cardiovasc Imaging 2017;18(12):1301-10.

71. Searns JB, Williams MC, MacBrayne CE, et al. Handshake antimicrobial stewardship as a model to recognize and prevent diagnostic errors. Diagnosis (Berl) 2020. https://doi.org/10.1515/dx-2020-0032. dx-2020-0032.

72. Filice GA, Drekonja DM, Thurn JR, et al. Diagnostic errors that lead to inappropriate antimicrobial Use. Infect Control Hosp Epidemiol 2015;36(8):949–56.
73. Goldman JL, Lee BR, Hersh AL, et al. Clinical diagnoses and antimicrobials predictive of pediatric antimicrobial stewardship recommendations: a program evaluation. Infect Control Hosp Epidemiol 2015;36(6):673–80.
74. Goldman JL, Newland JG, Price M, et al. Clinical impact of an antimicrobial stewardship program on high-risk pediatric patients. Infect Control Hosp Epidemiol 2019;40(9):968–73.
75. Carter SM, Rogers W, Heath I, et al. The challenge of overdiagnosis begins with its definition. BMJ 2015;350:h869. https://doi.org/10.1136/bmj.h869.
76. Jenniskens K, de Groot JAH, Reitsma JB, et al. Overdiagnosis across medical disciplines: a scoping review. BMJ Open 2017;7(12):e018448. https://doi.org/10.1136/bmjopen-2017-018448.
77. Boeckh M, Stevens-Ayers T, Travi G, et al. Cytomegalovirus (CMV) DNA quantitation in bronchoalveolar lavage fluid from Hematopoietic stem cell transplant Recipients with CMV pneumonia. J Infect Dis 2017;215(10):1514–22.
78. Bateman M, Oladele R, Kolls JK. Diagnosing Pneumocystis jirovecii pneumonia: a review of current methods and novel approaches. Med Mycol 2020;58(8):1015–28.
79. Wiener RS, Schwartz LM, Woloshin S. When a test is too good: how CT pulmonary angiograms find pulmonary emboli that do not need to be found. BMJ 2013;347: f3368. https://doi.org/10.1136/bmj.f3368.
80. Ehrman RR, Sullivan AN, Favot MJ, et al. Pathophysiology, echocardiographic evaluation, biomarker findings, and prognostic implications of septic cardiomyopathy: a review of the literature. Crit Care 2018;22(1):112.
81. Moynihan R, Heath I, Henry D. Selling sickness: the pharmaceutical industry and disease mongering. BMJ 2002;324(7342):886–91.
82. Pathirana T, Clark J, Moynihan R. Mapping the drivers of overdiagnosis to potential solutions. BMJ 2017;358:j3879. https://doi.org/10.1136/bmj.j3879.
83. Manja V, Guyatt G, You J, et al. Qualitative study of cardiologists' perceptions of factors influencing clinical practice decisions. Heart 2019;105(10):749–54.
84. Saini V, Garcia-Armesto S, Klemperer D, et al. Drivers of poor medical care. Lancet 2017;390(10090):178–90.
85. Blumenthal-Barby JS, Krieger H. Cognitive biases and heuristics in medical decision making: a critical review using a systematic search strategy. Med Decis Making 2015;35(4):539–57.
86. Hoffmann TC, Del Mar C. Clinicians' Expectations of the benefits and harms of treatments, screening, and tests: a systematic review. JAMA Intern Med 2017; 177(3):407–19.
87. Reddy K, Sinha P, O'Kane CM, et al. Subphenotypes in critical care: translation into clinical practice. Lancet Respir Med 2020;8(6):631–43.
88. Reilly JP, Calfee CS, Christie JD. Acute respiratory distress syndrome phenotypes. Semin Respir Crit Care Med 2019;40(1):19–30.
89. Annane D, Pastores SM, Rochwerg B, et al. Guidelines for the diagnosis and management of critical illness-related Corticosteroid insufficiency (CIRCI) in critically ill patients (Part I): society of critical care medicine (SCCM) and European society of intensive care medicine (ESICM) 2017. Crit Care Med 2017;45(12):2078–88.
90. Silver MJ, Li YH, Gragg LA, et al. Reduction of blood loss from diagnostic sampling in critically ill patients using a blood-conserving arterial line system. Chest 1993;104(6):1711–5.

Intensive Care Unit Decision-Making in Uncertain and Stressful Conditions Part 2
Cognitive Errors, Debiasing Strategies, and Enhancing Critical Thinking

Megan Christenson, MD, MPH, Anuj Shukla, MD, Jayshil J. Patel, MD*

KEYWORDS

- Diagnostic error • Cognitive error • Cognitive failure • Heuristics • Debiasing
- Critical thinking

KEY POINTS

- Cognitive failures are a common cause of diagnostic error and occur because of faulty thinking.
- System and individual based debiasing strategies to reduce diagnostic error have not been well studied in the critical care setting.
- Teaching critical thinking may prevent cognitive errors in a fast-paced, high acuity, and error prone setting such the intensive care unit.

INTRODUCTION

In 2015, the Institute of Medicine (now the National Academy of Medicine) labeled diagnostic error the blind spot of health care delivery.[1] A diagnostic error is defined as a "failure to develop an accurate explanation for a patient's health problem and/or failure to communicate that explanation." Autopsies, secondary reviews, and voluntary reports suggest diagnostic errors occur in up to 15% of cases, leading to adverse events in up to 90% of cases.

The intensive care unit (ICU) is a highly complex and fast-paced environment where patients necessitate time-sensitive management. History gathering and participation

Department of Medicine, Division of Pulmonary and Critical Care Medicine, Medical College of Wisconsin, Milwaukee, WI 53045, USA
* Corresponding author. 8701 West Watertown Plank Road, HUB, 8th Floor, Milwaukee, Wisconsin 53226, USA.
E-mail address: jpatel2@mcw.edu

Crit Care Clin 38 (2022) 89–101
https://doi.org/10.1016/j.ccc.2021.08.003
0749-0704/22/© 2021 Elsevier Inc. All rights reserved.

in physical examination are encumbered by mechanically ventilated, sedated, and unconscious or delirious patients. Multidisciplinary team members and consultants offer varying impressions. Critical care clinicians are often stabilizing patients, which leads to task switching between empirically treating and diagnosing. Thus, critical care physicians are vulnerable to diagnostic error.

These aforementioned factors create the perfect storm for the occurrence of diagnostic errors, which can have fatal consequences. In a retrospective study of 256 unplanned ICU admission, diagnostic errors were identified in 7%, and all errors were associated with harm.[2]

In this narrative review, the authors (1) describe why cognitive errors occur, (2) review the literature on the impact of system and individual level debiasing strategies on reducing such errors, and (3) outline a rationale and framework for teaching critical thinking.

WHY DO COGNITIVE ERRORS OCCUR?

Cognitive errors are a leading cause of diagnostic error and are faulty patterns of thinking.[3] In an analysis of 583 physician-reported diagnostic errors, a failure/delay in considering diagnosis, suboptimal weighing of information, or too much emphasis placed on competing diagnoses were the most common reasons for "what went wrong."[4] As a result, patients may be subject to unnecessary testing and incorrect therapies, which may lead to psychological/physical harm, toxicity, prolonged hospitalization, and even death.

To better understand cognitive errors, it is imperative to acknowledge the theory of clinical decision-making, which has *normative* and *descriptive* components. The normative component is "how decisions ideally *should be* made," whereas the descriptive is "how decisions *are actually* made." The normative component suggests decisions should be made using an analytical, or what behavioral economist Daniel Kahneman describes as system 2, mode of reasoning.[5] In approaching a diagnostic workup, such hypothetical-deductive reasoning includes incorporation of concepts such as pretest probability and likelihood ratios to determine likelihood of disease.

Pause here and see **Fig. 1**. *What is the answer?* Did you reach for your calculator? For most, the answer does not immediately come to mind. The task of multiplying large numbers requires forced attention. This example forces activation of system 2 thinking, which is deliberate, slow, and uses significant cognitive resources.[5] Stated differently, system 2 uses critical thinking skills.

Take another pause and look at **Fig. 2**. *Which emotion is displayed?* Did you intuitively identify happiness or joy? In effect, you were using what Kahneman describes as system 1 (reflexive) mode of thinking. This mode is hard-wired, fast, reflexive, requires minimal cognitive resource utilization (compared with system 2), and relies on pattern recognition. System 1 uses *heuristics* or "rules of thumb."[5] Heuristics are necessary because thinking carefully, analyzing, and using hypothetical-deductive reasoning at each patient encounter is cognitively exhausting and inefficient, which may lead to errors from "overthinking" or "analysis paralysis." However, it is often an overreliance on system 1 that leads to cognitive failures/errors and subsequent diagnostic errors.

Recall, cognitive errors are faults in assessment or synthesis of information. There are many types of cognitive errors in medicine. Consider this example:

What is 179 multiplied by 491?

Fig. 1. An example of system 2 activation.

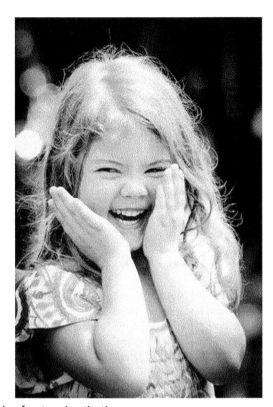

Fig. 2. An example of system 1 activation.

You are taking hand-off in a busy ICU. Your colleague informs you that Mr. Smith is a 50-year old "frequent flyer" who has a history of severe systolic heart failure and poorly controlled hypertension who presented again with shortness of breath that is, being managed as decompensated heart failure. His blood pressure is 90/50 mm Hg and has a temperature of 100° F. You go and evaluate him at the start of your shift and notice he awake and alert but tachypneic and hypoxemic with new 8 L oxygen requirement. He has no lung crackles and JVD is absent. His skin is warm with bounding pulses. Chest radiograph is reported by the radiologist as "could be consistent with heart failure" and EKG shows sinus tachycardia. You're called to a rapid floor transfer. You decide to continue diuresis for Mr. Smith.

Take a moment and consider the elements of this case that will promote cognitive errors:

(1) Hand-off medicine and "framing" the patient as a "frequent flyer" may promote *anchoring* or a tendency to be unduly persuaded by features encountered early in a patient presentation of illness.

(2) Anchoring onto a diagnosis may lead to *premature closure*, where one settles on a diagnosis without enough evidence or without carefully considering contradictory information. This patient has a fever and has a low blood pressure for someone who has poorly controlled hypertension.

(3) Despite the low-grade temperature, lower blood pressure, and absence of lung crackles, the chest radiograph could be used to confirm a handed-off diagnosis. This phenomenon is *confirmation bias*, in which one only observes aspects of the case one was "primed" to see, which "confirms" the established diagnosis.

(4) Finally, the competing duty of managing other sick patients may determine one's cognitive and affective states and predispose to cognitive errors. Other situational factors such as fatigue, lack of sleep, and past experiences shape our clinical decision-making (collectively known as cognitive dispositions to respond).[4,6]

STRATEGIES TO REDUCE COGNITIVE ERRORS

The National Academies of Science, Engineering, and Medicine published a set of 8 goals for reducing diagnostic error (**Table 1**).[1] Intensive care physicians are optimally positioned to promote a culture of diagnostic safety using system-based and individual strategies to reduce cognitive errors specifically (**Table 2**). In this section, the authors examine these strategies.

SYSTEMS-BASED STRATEGIES TO REDUCE COGNITIVE ERRORS
Checklists

Checklists are frequently used in the ICU setting because they have been shown to be effective at preventing harm. Pronovost and colleagues[7] showed that catheter-related bloodstream infections could be reduced by clinicians adopting 5 evidence-based procedures on a checklist. Ely and colleagues[8] suggested 3 types of checklists could be used to reduce diagnostic error: (1) a general checklist for a diagnosis, (2) a checklist of differential diagnosis to reduce premature closure, and (3) a checklist that serves as a cognitive forcing function.[8] The third checklist rules out life-threatening diagnoses for a particular set of symptoms or to ensure all critical elements of a correct procedure were followed. Sibbald demonstrated checklists directed at interpretation of an electrocardiogram (ECG) resulted in a small but consistent reduction in diagnostic error at all learner levels, with the greatest benefit in novices.[9] In a follow-up study comparing debiasing checklists with knowledge retrieval checklists to reduce

Table 1 National Academies of Sciences, Engineering, and Medicine: goals for improving diagnosis and reducing diagnostic error	
Goal 1	Facilitate More Effective Teamwork in the Diagnostic Process Among Health Care Professionals, Patients, and their families
Goal 2	Enhance health care professional education and training in the diagnostic process
Goal 3	Ensure that health information technologies support patients and health care professionals in the diagnostic process
Goal 4	Develop and deploy approaches to identify, learn from, and reduce diagnostic errors and near misses in clinical practice
Goal 5	Establish a work system and culture that supports the diagnostic process and improvements in diagnostic performance
Goal 6	Develop a reporting environment and medical liability system that facilitates improved diagnosis by learning from diagnostic errors and near misses
Goal 7	Design a payment and care delivery environment that supports the diagnostic process
Goal 8	Provide dedicated funding for research on the diagnostic process and diagnostic errors

Table 2
Common cognitive biases

Common Cognitive Biases	Description
Anchoring	Holding onto a diagnosis early in the diagnostic process while ignoring incoming contradictory evidence
Availability	Accepting diagnoses based on features of a case that readily come to mind
Confirmation	Tendency to look for confirmative evidence for a diagnosis, rather than evidence to refute it
Diagnostic momentum	Attaching diagnostic labels to cases and excluding other possibilities once attached
Framing effect	Presenting a case in a way that influences the diagnosis
Premature closure	Failure to consider alternative diagnoses after an initial diagnosis is made

diagnostic error related to ECG interpretation, Sibbald and colleagues found no advantage of using a checklist for identifying specific aspects of an ECG or to identify cognitive biases.[10] In a systematic review of strategies to reduce diagnostic error, Abimanyi-Ochom and colleagues[11] found 4 studies that tested the efficacy of checklists in reducing diagnostic error and concluded that checklists could prevent diagnostic errors because checklists include additional diagnostic possibilities. Unfortunately, these studies were not conducted in an ICU setting, and their impact on reducing diagnostic error in an ICU setting remains unknown.

Decision Support Tools

Decision support tools have been shown to improve diagnostic accuracy for a variety of conditions[11–13] and could be used to quickly establish common diagnoses. Decision support tools are already implemented in several settings to promote evidence-based use of imaging and/or laboratory tests to reduce costs.[11] In a systematic review, Abimanyi-Ochom and colleagues identified 11 studies of computerized decision support systems to reduce diagnostic error and found support systems enhanced pediatric diagnoses in junior physicians, increased accuracy in diagnosing the cause of acute abdominal pain, and provided more accurate prediction of Alzheimer disease.[8] Computer-aided support systems enhanced time to small bowel obstruction diagnosis, as compared with radiology (1 hour vs 16 hours).[8] Computer-aided radiology interpretation, as compared with single radiologist interpretation, was found in one study to enhance diagnostic accuracy.[8] These findings, although not specific to ICU patients, remain relevant because patients with bowel obstruction require ICU level care and ICU patients, in general, often undergo extensive imaging.

Metacognitive Strategies

Metacognitive strategies reflect on how failures of the system can contribute to diagnostic error. Examples include bedside teaching, morbidity and mortality (M&M) conference, and case conferences. These venues serve as opportunities to point out system-level factors that were implicated in a delayed or missed diagnosis.[14] Reason's Swiss Cheese Model has been used to identify the root cause of medical error.[15] One institution showed that M&M conferences that focused on how systemic failures contributed to medical error increased awareness of system-based practice and led to improvements in patient care.[16] It is imperative that any strategy that focuses on cognitive failures also include the interplay between systemic factors that play a role in diagnostic error.

INDIVIDUAL EDUCATIONAL STRATEGIES TO REDUCE COGNITIVE ERROR
Teaching the Diagnostic Process and Heuristics

Intuitively, education to generate awareness of the diagnostic process would be the first step in preventing faulty information synthesis. However, studies that have evaluated teaching system 1 and 2 modes of thinking have not proved their efficacy enhancing diagnostic accuracy.[3,17] Numerous studies have tested whether creating awareness of cognitive biases could reduce diagnostic errors. In a study evaluating the impact of a cognitive bias curriculum in internal medicine residents, Reilly and colleagues found the intervention group identified biases on a written test and on a video scenario.[18] In a study that taught emergency medicine residents cognitive biases, Bond and colleagues found emergency medicine residents perceived they had learned about biases.[19] Unfortunately, in both studies, the effect of cognitive bias education on diagnostic error reduction was not tested. Three studies evaluating the effect of cognitive bias education on diagnostic error found no difference.[3] These studies were conducted in internal medicine, family medicine, and emergency medicine trainees, and the effect of the intervention in an ICU setting is unknown.

Relational Reasoning

Relational reasoning can be described as *strategies to identify meaningful patterns from a large body of information,* which can serve to mitigate faulty synthesis.[20] Relational reasoning can be used to learn and process information in many fields including medical education and the ICU. In fact, it seems that strong problem solvers in the medical field already use some of these techniques described later to arrive at a diagnosis.[21] The concepts of relational reasoning have been studied and applied to the fields of science, mathematics, and engineering[22–25]; however, there has been sparse data regarding the use of relational reasoning in undergraduate and graduate medical education. Dumas and colleagues[20] argue that "relational reasoning strategies help clinicians to be metacognitive about their own clinical reasoning and these processes can be harnessed to use in clinical reasoning instruction."

Table 3
Relational reasoning strategies explained with clinical examples

Characteristic	Relationship	Clinical Example
Analogy	Similarity	Describing alveoli like balloons that require force to inhale but have elastic recoil that assists in exhalation
Anomaly	Discrepancy	A patient being treated for septic shock is found to have a large drop in hemoglobin
Antinomy	Incompatibility	In a patient with no prior heparin exposure, thrombocytopenia at day 2 of admission cannot be heparin-induced thrombocytopenia based on our understanding of pathophysiology
Antithesis	Opposition	In a patient with endocarditis, the infectious disease team is advocating for valve surgery, whereas the cardiothoracic surgery team believes medical management with intravenous antibiotics will suffice

Adapted from Dumas D, Torre DM, Durning SJ. Using Relational Reasoning Strategies to Help Improve Clinical Reasoning Practice. Acad Med. 2018;93(5):709-714; with permission.

Alexander and colleagues[26] described 4 characteristics of relational reasoning that can apply to diagnostic reasoning: *analogy*, *anomaly*, *antinomy*, and *antithesis* (**Table 3**). Relational reasoning can be interrelated with cognitive biases. *Analogy* could be subject to availability bias when a clinician compares their current patient with bradycardia with their previous patient who ended up having a cerebral herniation. If the same clinician dismisses *anomalies*, such as their patient's history of heart disease and use of a beta-blocker, the clinician may be susceptible to premature closure. Failing to use *anomaly* could also put a clinician at risk for confirmation bias, in which they only look for clinical features of the case that support their diagnosis.

In the same example, the clinician could use *antinomy* to lower the likelihood of cerebral herniation when they conclude that the patient does not have any focal neurologic deficits on examination. The clinician, in this example, could be subject to anchoring bias. Lack of *antithesis* in clinical decision-making could promote diagnostic momentum where the initial diagnosis is accepted and unchallenged despite contradictory evidence. Lack of *antithesis* could also lead to bandwagon effect, where other treatment regimens that may be better for the patient are not suggested in favor of the opinion of the senior member of the team.[27]

Horizontal and Vertical Tracing

Shimizu[28] proposed horizonal and vertical tracing to improve diagnostic accuracy by identifying a primary condition or disease and ascertaining comorbidities and underlying conditions that support the diagnosis. Horizontal tracing involves visualizing conditions that are likely to occur together with a primary condition. For example, when a clinician considers the diagnosis of giant cell arteritis, they should look for concurrent polymyalgia rheumatica. Vertical tracing identifies a primary diagnosis and looks for an underlying diagnosis that could explain this primary diagnosis. For example, in an ICU patient who presents with acute hypoxemic respiratory failure, an underlying diagnosis (such as a hematologic cancer, which predisposes a patient to be immunocompromised) that contributes to the primary diagnosis must be discovered. In the ICU case, the clinician considers a differential diagnosis of infectious pneumonia, pulmonary embolism, aspiration event, or varying forms of pulmonary edema, which contributes to the underlying hypoxemia. Shimizu proposes that horizontal and vertical tracing can reduce the cognitive workload and may decrease the chance of missing (or otherwise overlooked) diagnoses to facilitate rapid identification of the correct diagnosis.[28] Unfortunately, studies evaluating the efficacy of horizontal and vertical tracing in an ICU setting are lacking.

Cognitive Forcing Strategies and Metacognition

Cognitive forcing is a promising debiasing strategy, although the utility and effectiveness has yet to take hold in broader clinical practice. Cognitive forcing strategies (CFS) work by applying a form of self-monitoring, or metacognitive training, during clinical decision-making. This form of self-reflection may be achieved by acknowledging the risk for error, potential biases that may influence clinical decision-making, and actively using a cognitive strategy to counteract a potential bias. To date, a paucity of observational and randomized controlled trials (RCTs) has evaluated the effectiveness in CFS in minimizing diagnostic errors. Sherbino and colleagues[29] evaluated cognitive forcing strategies in a case series with fourth-year medical students after an emergency medicine rotation, specifically teaching search satisfying bias and availability bias. The students were given case vignettes to evaluate for primary and secondary diagnoses, as well as the generalizability of transfer among cases. They found that despite having formal instruction on CFS, fewer than half of the students used CFS to debias. In addition, there was lack of transfer with the CFS that were forgotten over time.[29]

Mamede and colleagues[30] and Coderre and colleagues[31] evaluated metacognitive training in the form of self-reflection among internal medicine residents. Mamede and colleagues found that cognitive reflection decreased the tendency toward availability bias.[30] Coderre and colleagues found that reflection on initial diagnoses, particularly initial inaccurate diagnoses, was helpful and did not lead to new errors if the initial diagnoses were correct.[31] However, neither study was conducted in actual clinical practice.

Two randomized control trials have evaluated CFS using mnemonic techniques to help physician trainees. Wolpaw and colleagues[32] randomized third-year medical students to the SNAPPS (Summarize history and findings, Narrow the differential; Analyze the differential; Probe preceptor about uncertainties; Plan management; Select case-related issues for self-study) technique, compared with a group with direct feedback from preceptors and a usual-and-customary group (control group). They found that the students who used the SNAPPS technique were more likely to correct flawed reasoning, reduce diagnostic and therapeutic errors, and express uncertainties more often than the other groups. However, the outcome measurements did not focus on accuracy of diagnoses, but rather on the reasoning process itself. O'Sullivan and colleagues[33] used the mnemonic SLOW (Sure?, Look/lack/link, Opposite, Worst case scenario) and randomized medical students, residents, and attendings to use the SLOW mnemonic versus standard of care in case vignette questions designed to trigger particular biases. In the intervention group, the physicians and trainees were prompted on the SLOW mnemonic before and after cases and were asked to complete an onscreen checklist prompted by the SLOW tool. The primary outcome was the number of correct responses to case vignettes. They found no significant difference in the number of correct responses between groups. However, the qualitative effects were positive, as more physicians and trainees found CFS helpful in improving quality of thought and problem-solving skills.

Group Decision-Making and Feedback

The propensity toward error and cognitive biases are more common during high stress, time-intensive, and high-acuity situations,[34] which in an ICU setting could represent a large portion of the day. Thus, recognizing when one might be prone to cognitive bias is important, and an ICU provider should consider a broad differential or identify anomalies to prevent error. Strategies to seek a broad differential include democratizing ICU rounds, whereby members of a multidisciplinary team provide opinions, especially during times of uncertainty.[35] Providing real-time feedback on components of diagnostic reasoning and decision-making can serve as a CFS, which may enhance diagnostic accuracy.[36–38] In a study assessing the impact of group decision-making in 10 trauma scenarios among 83 surgical, emergency medicine, and anesthesia residents, Murray and colleagues found group decision-making led to higher performance scores when managing heuristic-based scenarios. Group decision-making remains a fruitful possibility for reducing errors, but further studies in an ICU setting are needed.

LIMITATIONS TO DEBIASING STRATEGIES

Clinical decisions depend on numerous factors including the level of the learner and factors related to the clinical learning environment. For example, physicians who have deliberately practiced medicine with a rich understanding of the diagnostic process may be more likely to incorporate system 1 thinking when arriving at a diagnosis. Over a period of many years, they have acquired more complete illness scripts (prototypical understanding of a disease), and debiasing strategies may be an inherent component of their repertoire for arriving at a diagnosis. On the contrary, physicians in training, who may be unaware of the diagnostic process, and "how they think" may benefit from explicit use of CFS. Therefore, standardizing debiasing strategies may not be feasible. Furthermore, the evidence basis of educational strategies directed at reducing errors is largely negative and limited to observational and small RCT level data. Furthermore, many debiasing strategies have been conducted in mock practice settings, which limits interpretation and extrapolation to real-time practice. Finally, system level factors, such as patient complexity, increasing clinical workload, and a continual push for efficiency may limit implementation of cognitive debiasing strategies (at a systems level).

TEACHING CRITICAL THINKING IN THE INTENSIVE CARE UNIT

The authors have presented systems-based and individual debiasing strategies aimed at reducing diagnostic errors. Unfortunately, as outlined earlier, implementing individual strategies have not been shown to universally enhance diagnostic accuracy nor reduce errors. However, these strategies are considered integral components of critical thinking, which is defined as "the ability to apply higher cognitive skills and/or the disposition to be deliberative about thinking that leads to action that is, logical and appropriate."[39] Higher cognitive skills include analysis, synthesis, self-reflection,

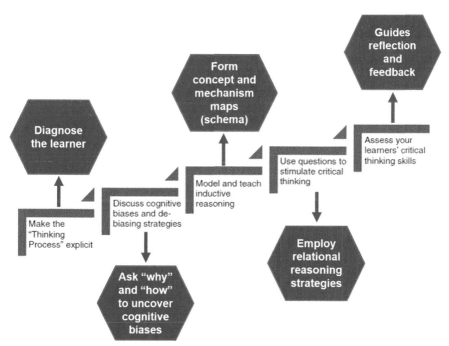

Fig. 3. Framework for critical thinking in the ICU. (*Adapted from* Hayes MM, Chatterjee S, Schwartzstein RM. Critical Thinking in Critical Care: Five Strategies to Improve Teaching and Learning in the Intensive Care Unit. Ann Am Thorac Soc. 2017;14(4):569 to 575. https://doi.org/10.1513/AnnalsATS.201612-1009AS; with permission.)

and perspective taking.[39] A complex environment as the ICU increases the risk for cognitive failure, thus critical thinking is crucial. Evidence to guide best educational practices and consensus on optimal methods to teach critical thinking are lacking. Hayes and colleagues have outlined a 5-step framework for explicitly teaching critical thinking in the ICU by using methods that (1) optimize the ability to diagnose the learner, (2) enhance learner engagement and development, (3) recognize and provide feedback on cognitive biases, and (4) promote metacognition (**Fig. 3**).[40]

Strategy 1 is explicating the thinking process. Instead of passively listening to an assessment and plan, the attending physician asks "how" and "why" questions to get an understanding of where the learner operates on Bloom's taxonomy. For example, in an immunocompromised patient presenting with acute hypoxemic respiratory failure who has a lung infiltrate, asking "why" the learner thinks the patient has infectious pneumonia gauges the learner's level of understanding (diagnose the learner).

Strategy 2 is to point-out and teach cognitive biases and debiasing strategies. In the same immunocompromised patient who presents with acute hypoxemic respiratory failure and has a lung infiltrate, asking "why" may reveal an opportunity to uncover lurking availability and/or confirmation bias.[40]

Strategy 3 is to model and teach inductive reasoning. Hypothetico-deductive reasoning involves forming differential diagnoses (the hypotheses), which are matched to facts obtained from the history and physical. The best match is often the answer. Inductive reasoning uses a few data points to generate hypotheses based on anatomic or pathophysiologic constructs. For example, in a patient with thrombocytopenia, the mechanisms for low platelets are (a) increased destruction, (b) sequestration, or (c) decreased production. Inductive reasoning allows the learner to generate diagnostic schema or systematic approaches to a problem, which allows consideration of broad differential diagnoses.[39,40]

Strategy 4 uses questions to stimulate critical thinking. Hayes and colleagues suggest it is important to avoid "quiz show" type questions that test whether a trainee can recall facts. Instead, asking questions that challenge the learner to explicate their thinking are informative to diagnose the learner. Cognitive forcing and relational reasoning strategies can be used at this step. For example, in the same

Table 4	
Milestones of critical thinking and the hallmark of each stage	
Critical Thinking Milestone	**Hallmark**
Challenged thinker[a]	Environmental pressures such as time forces thinkers to make rapid decisions (system 1 thinking) where cognitive biases such as premature closure is common
Unreflective thinker	Narrow differential, cognitive biases common
Beginning critical thinker	Broad differential without relational reasoning, cognitive biases common
Practicing critical thinker	Broad but unweighted differential based on mechanistic thinking (inductive reasoning)
Advanced critical thinker	Broad differential, admits uncertainty, engages in metacognition, and solicits feedback

[a] Any thinker can be challenged due to environmental pressures or time constraints.

Papp KK, Huang GC, Lauzon Clabo LM, et al. Milestones of critical thinking: a developmental model for medicine and nursing. Acad Med 2014;89:715–20.

immunocompromised patient with acute hypoxemic respiratory failure and a lung infiltrate, asking "Why do you think the patient has infectious pneumonia?" is likely to open a window into the learner's thought process, and following up with questions such as "What components of the patient's history do not fit?" serves as checkpoints.[40]

Strategy 5 is to assess the learner's critical thinking.[40] For learners to remain engaged and become, as Hayes and colleagues call, "challenged critical thinkers," educators assess critical thinking by reviewing milestones of critical thinking (**Table 4**).[40,41] For example, asking a learner "How are you doing with the new admission?" and "How are you thinking about the case?" can uncover a learner's level of critical thinking. In the case of the immunocompromised patient with acute hypoxemic respiratory failure with a lung infiltrate, a learner acknowledging a working diagnosis of infectious pneumonia but expressing uncertainty given components of the case that do not fit (using relational reasoning strategies) and acknowledging barriers to the diagnostic process (eg, time constraints, other patient related duties) is reflective of a practicing critical thinker.

SUMMARY

Cognitive failures are a common cause of diagnostic errors in medicine. Cognitive debiasing strategies, although intuitive, have not been borne out by the evidence to be wholly effective in reducing cognitive failures. The evidentiary base is composed of observational and small RCTs, many conducted in the emergency department and in the general medicine ward, which limits extrapolation to an ICU setting. Efficacy data for debiasing strategies in an ICU setting are lacking. Moreover, based on the fast-paced nature of an ICU, time-constraints, and ambiguity in clinical practice, it is unclear whether errors are entirely preventable.[3] Nonetheless, until further research can inform best educational practices, teaching critical thinking that incorporates a combination of explicit thinking, recognizing, and providing feedback on cognitive biases, using inductive reasoning, using relational reasoning, and assessing learner skills may be valuable for learner assessment and development, as well as for reducing diagnostic error.

CONFLICTS OF INTEREST

All authors have no conflicts of interest to disclose.

REFERENCES

1. Committee on Diagnostic Error in Health Care, Board on Health Care Services, Institute of Medicine, The National Academies of Sciences, Engineering, and Medicine. In: Balogh EP, Miller BT, Ball JR, editors. Improving diagnosis in health care. Washington (DC): National Academies Press (US); 2015.
2. Bergl PA, Taneja A, El-Kareh R, et al. Frequency, risk factors, causes, and Consequences of diagnostic errors in critically Ill medical patients: a retrospective Cohort study. Crit Care Med 2019;47(11):e902–10.
3. Norman GR, Monteiro SD, Sherbino J, et al. The causes of errors in clinical reasoning: cognitive biases, knowledge deficits, and dual process thinking. Acad Med 2017;92(1):23–30.
4. Schiff GD, Hasan O, Kim S, et al. Diagnostic error in medicine: analysis of 583 physician-reported errors. Arch Intern Med 2009;169(20):1881–7.

5. Kahneman D. Thinking fast and slow. New York: Farrar, Strauss, and Giroux; 2011.
6. Croskerry P. Diagnostic failure: a cognitive and affective approach. In: Henriksen K, Battles JB, Marks ES, et al, editors. Advances in patient safety: from research to implementation. vol. 2. Rockville (MD): Concepts and Methodology; 2005.
7. Pronovost P, Needham D, Berenholtz S, et al. An intervention to decrease catheter-related bloodstream infections in the ICU. N Engl J Med 2006;355(26): 2725–32.
8. Ely JW, Graber ML, Croskerry P. Checklists to reduce diagnostic errors. Acad Med 2011;86(3):307–13.
9. Sibbald M, De Bruin AB, van Merrienboer JJ. Finding and fixing mistakes: do checklists work for clinicians with different levels of experience? Adv Health Sci Educ Theor Pract 2014;19(1):43–51.
10. Sibbald M, Sherbino J, Ilgen JS, et al. Debiasing versus knowledge retrieval checklists to reduce diagnostic error in ECG interpretation. Adv Health Sci Educ Theor Pract 2019;24(3):427–40.
11. Abimanyi-Ochom J, Bohingamu Mudiyanselage S, Catchpool M, et al. Strategies to reduce diagnostic errors: a systematic review. BMC Med Inform Decis Mak 2019;19(1):174.
12. Barnett GO, Cimino JJ, Hupp JA, et al. An evolving diagnostic decision-support system. JAMA 1987;258(1):67–74.
13. Ramnarayan P, Roberts GC, Coren M, et al. Assessment of the potential impact of a reminder system on the reduction of diagnostic errors: a quasi-experimental study. BMC Med Inform Decis Mak 2006;6:22.
14. Trowbridge RL, Dhaliwal G, Cosby KS. Educational agenda for diagnostic error reduction. BMJ Qual Saf 2013;22(Suppl 2):ii28–32.
15. Reason J. Human error: models and management. BMJ 2000;320(7237):768–70.
16. Szostek JH, Wieland ML, Loertscher LL, et al. A systems approach to morbidity and mortality conference. Am J Med 2010;123(7):663–8.
17. Norman G, Sherbino J, Dore K, et al. The etiology of diagnostic errors: a controlled trial of system 1 versus system 2 reasoning. Acad Med 2014;89(2): 277–84.
18. Reilly JB, Ogdie AR, Von Feldt JM, et al. Teaching about how doctors think: a longitudinal curriculum in cognitive bias and diagnostic error for residents. BMJ Qual Saf 2013;22(12):1044–50.
19. Bond WF, Deitrick LM, Arnold DC, et al. Using simulation to instruct emergency medicine residents in cognitive forcing strategies. Acad Med 2004;79(5):438–46.
20. Dumas D, Torre DM, Durning SJ. Using relational reasoning strategies to help improve clinical reasoning practice. Acad Med 2018;93(5):709–14.
21. Patel VL, Evans DA, Kaufman DR. Reasoning strategies and the use of biomedical knowledge by medical students. Med Educ 1990;24(2):129–36.
22. Richland LE, Simms N. Analogy, higher order thinking, and education. Wiley Interdiscip Rev Cogn Sci 2015;6(2):177–92.
23. Murphy PK, Firetto CM, Greene JA. Enriching students' Scientific thinking through relational reasoning: Seeking evidence in Texts, tasks, and Talk. Educ Psychol Rev 2017;29(1):105–17.
24. Chan J, Schunn C. The impact of analogies on creative concept generation: lessons from an in vivo study in engineering design. Cogn Sci 2015;39(1):126–55.
25. Dumas D. Relational reasoning in science, medicine, and engineering. Educ Psychol Rev 2017;29(1):73–95.

26. Alexander PA. The Disciplined reading and learning research L. Reading into the Future: Competence for the 21st Century. Educ Psychol 2012;47(4):259–80.
27. Whelehan DF, Conlon KC, Ridgway PF. Medicine and heuristics: cognitive biases and medical decision-making. Ir J Med Sci 2020;189(4):1477–84.
28. Shimizu T. Horizontal and vertical tracing: a cognitive forcing strategy to improve diagnostic accuracy. Postgrad Med J 2020;96(1140):581–3.
29. Sherbino J, Yip S, Dore KL, et al. The effectiveness of cognitive forcing strategies to decrease diagnostic error: an exploratory study. Teach Learn Med 2011;23(1): 78–84.
30. Mamede S, van Gog T, van den Berge K, et al. Effect of availability bias and reflective reasoning on diagnostic accuracy among internal medicine residents. Jama 2010;304(11):1198–203.
31. Coderre S, Wright B, McLaughlin K. To think is good: querying an initial hypothesis reduces diagnostic error in medical students. Acad Med 2010;85(7):1125–9.
32. Wolpaw T, Papp KK, Bordage G. Using SNAPPS to facilitate the expression of clinical reasoning and uncertainties: a randomized comparison group trial. Acad Med 2009;84(4):517–24.
33. O'Sullivan ED, Schofield SJ. A cognitive forcing tool to mitigate cognitive bias - a randomised control trial. BMC Med Educ 2019;19(1):12.
34. Garrouste Orgeas M, Timsit JF, Soufir L, et al. Impact of adverse events on outcomes in intensive care unit patients. Crit Care Med 2008;36(7):2041–7.
35. Croskerry P, Singhal G, Mamede S. Cognitive debiasing 2: impediments to and strategies for change. BMJ Qual Saf 2013;22(Suppl 2):ii65–72.
36. Yulei J, Robert MN, Robert AS, et al. Relative gains in diagnostic accuracy between computer-aided diagnosis and independent double reading. Paper presented at: Proc.SPIE2000.
37. Elstein AS. Thinking about diagnostic thinking: a 30-year perspective. Adv Health Sci Educ Theor Pract 2009;14(Suppl 1):7–18.
38. de Wet C, Black C, Luty S, et al. Implementation of the trigger review method in Scottish general practices: patient safety outcomes and potential for quality improvement. BMJ Qual Saf 2017;26(4):335–42.
39. Richards JB, Hayes MM, Schwartzstein RM. Teaching clinical reasoning and critical thinking: from cognitive theory to practical Application. Chest 2020;158(4): 1617–28.
40. Hayes MM, Chatterjee S, Schwartzstein RM. Critical thinking in critical care: five strategies to improve teaching and learning in the intensive care Unit. Ann Am Thorac Soc 2017;14(4):569–75.
41. Papp KK, Huang GC, Lauzon Clabo LM, et al. Milestones of critical thinking: a developmental model for medicine and nursing. Acad Med 2014;89(5):715–20.

Learning from Missed Opportunities Through Reflective Practice

Gopi J. Astik, MD, MS[a,*], Andrew P.J. Olson, MD[b]

KEYWORDS

- Diagnostic error • Reflection • Case review • Learning

KEY POINTS

- Identification of errors and missed opportunities is only the first step in the learning process.
- Analysis of cases can be conducted in various ways through multiple modalities and tools.
- Reflective practice surrounding diagnostic decisions is imperative for learning and growth.

INTRODUCTION

People improve performance by learning from their own experiences and identifying how a decision or action made at one point in time influences an outcome. This learning cycle begins with an experience followed by reflection, abstraction, and planning for future actions.[1] This critical appraisal of one's decisions and their impact is one form of reflection, and reflective practice is found across many fields of human performance, including medicine.

DEFINITIONS

Reflection can take 2 major forms: reflection *on* action, in which a person looks back on a decision or event and considers how the decision, its underlying processes, and the context in which it was made all impact an outcome; and refection *in* action, in which a person is able to consider these factors in near–real-time to modify a decision to improve an outcome. It can be helpful to consider reflection on action as aimed at improving future decisions and outcomes, while reflection in action is focused on improving a current decision. Both reflection in action and reflection on action are fundamental for improving performance, yet standard processes to enable—or at least not inhibit—this reflection about diagnostic performance are lacking in medicine

[a] Division of Hospital Medicine, Northwestern University Feinberg School of Medicine, 211 East Ontario Street, Suite 1300, Chicago, IL 60611, USA; [b] Department of Medicine and Pediatrics, University of Minnesota Medical School, 420 Delaware Street SE, MMC 284, Minneapolis, MN 55455, USA
* Corresponding author.
E-mail address: gastik@nm.org

Crit Care Clin 38 (2022) 103–112
https://doi.org/10.1016/j.ccc.2021.09.003
0749-0704/22/© 2021 Elsevier Inc. All rights reserved.

today.[2] When combined with the reality that there is an unacceptable number of missed opportunities to make an accurate and timely diagnosis and harms related to these diagnostic errors, the lack of systematic mechanisms to enable and ensure reflection about diagnostic reasoning is especially problematic. However, there are recent advances in understanding diagnostic errors (ie, missed opportunities to make a diagnosis) as well as reflection in medicine.

DISCUSSION

Diagnosis can be viewed as both the process used to arrive at an explanation for a patient's health problem or that explanation itself, and reflection serves an important role in improving both diagnostic processes and outcomes.[3] However, operationalizing this reflection can be challenging and requires an intentional design to ensure that reflection can actually occur effectively. Said differently, there is no doubt that both reflection *on* action and *in* action are important and likely effective at improving performance, so there must be a reason that processes to support reflection regarding diagnosis in medicine do not presently exist.

The reality is that medicine has, in general, relied on a fundamentally flawed assumption: that "no news is good news." We assume that our patients, their families, their care team, or our colleagues will inform us when one of our diagnoses was in error so that we cannot make the same error again. Yet, this assumption has been proven to be incorrect time and again; in turn, clinicians generally are not used to receiving feedback about their diagnostic reasoning and are usually overconfident in their abilities because they do not receive this feedback.[4] Thus, there exists an urgent need to develop, implement, and evaluate systematic approaches to enable, support, and ensure that reflection in the midst of, and about, diagnoses can occur.[5]

Learning from Diagnostic Errors

An important first step to improve diagnostic practice through reflection is to identify which cases up which to reflect, both in real-time and as part of a larger, retrospective program of reflective practice. Although it might be ideal to have mechanisms to reflect on all cases, this arrangement is impractical for most clinicians given the volume of their clinical practice. Systems to aggregate outcomes to allow an individual clinician to glean lessons from their overall body of cases are in early development.[6] Instead, most efforts have been aimed at identifying cases from which substantive learning is most likely to occur and thus future practice be improved. These cases are often those in which a missed opportunity to make a diagnosis—that is, a diagnostic error—has occurred. However, it should be noted that programs of reflection should also seek to include cases whereby diagnostic excellence occurred; that is, we can also learn from being right.

This first step is often the hardest because it requires identification of a missed opportunity, and these missed opportunities can occur either as a missed opportunity in a process (with or without an attendant poor outcome), a poor outcome, or both.[7] When considering cases to analyze, it is important to recognize that good diagnostic process does not always lead to good diagnostic outcomes, nor does a flawed diagnostic process always lead to poor diagnostic outcomes. Take, for example, a patient who has a CT of the chest ordered to evaluate for pulmonary embolism in whom a dissecting thoracic aortic aneurysm is found. The correct diagnosis was made (perhaps serendipitously) despite the clinician suspecting a different and ultimately incorrect condition. Thus, it is generally important to reflect on both the diagnostic outcome (ie, the correct label) and process to arrive at that label.

However, the recognition of errors alone is not sufficient to improve performance. Event reporting systems rely on active reporting of a problem or change. If an error is recognized, the next step involves reporting the error by someone involved. This usually requires extra time to document along with the possibility of self-incrimination and future consequences. Once errors are reported, there is often little feedback on changes or updates which further prevents future reporting.

One common mechanism by which cases to review is identified in patient safety work is through the incident or adverse event reporting systems. These systems are an important and deeply ingrained solution by which incidents are systematically captured for analysis in modern health care settings. Incident or event reporting systems, however, have been somewhat unreliable in identifying diagnostic errors; this lack of reliability likely relates to the longitudinal and dynamic nature of the diagnostic process, low physician adverse event reporting rates in general, and suboptimal recognition of diagnostic errors.[3,8] Studies have shown a minority of errors are reported via incident reporting systems for many of the reasons previously mentioned.[9] However, many institutions have implemented new or enhanced adverse event reporting systems that more reliably capture diagnostic errors.[8] Studies have attempted to improve incident reporting by using abbreviated electronic reporting methods with some positive results, although the long-term impact remains unknown.[10] Others have shown reporting cases as a diagnostic "learning opportunity" rather than an "error" yielded increased reporting.[11]

In addition to adverse event reporting systems, there has been substantial interest in identifying reliable and scalable strategies to identify diagnostic errors using electronic health record (EHR)-based triggers, as has been shown to be effective in identifying other quality and safety events.[12,13] Trigger tools seek to identify signals that indicate an adverse event using data in the EHR to allow further analysis and reflection on cases; examples specific to diagnostic error might include unplanned return visits to an emergency department, clinical deterioration requiring rescue care, or unexpected in-hospital deaths. EHR-based triggers for identifying diagnostic errors are an area of intense study, although significant challenges remain given the complexity of diagnostic information, the dynamic nature of the diagnostic process, the unpredictable sensitivity of triggers for identifying errors, and the varied methods by which the diagnostic process is documented in the EHR. However, implementable and accessible trigger tools for diagnostic safety are becoming more prevalent as their evidence base expands.[14,15]

There are other important means by which cases may be identified on which clinicians and teams can reflect to improve diagnosis in future cases. These involve peer-review systems, traditional morbidity and mortality conferences (MMCs), case conferences, as well as many others.

Approach: How to Analyze Cases for Learning and Improvement

Once cases in which there is a suggestion that the diagnostic process or outcome could have been improved (that is, a diagnostic error may have occurred), formal processes must be developed to analyze these cases to enable reflection and maximize learning.[6] There are many tools used to retrospectively review medical records which assist with evaluation for diagnostic errors in different ways. It should be noted that many of these tools were developed primarily as research tools for studying diagnostic errors; however, they have an application to seeking to improve diagnosis in the clinical environment by enabling robust and standard case analysis. The SaferDx and Revised SaferDx tools created by Singh and colleagues consist of objective criteria to assess for the presence of diagnostic errors.[16,17] Through a series of questions, the reviewer is asked to assess the diagnostic process including patient history, testing, examination, and plan to eventually decide whether a diagnostic error did occur. This tool has been validated for use in outpatient and inpatient settings and applied to both adult and pediatric patients.[16,18] This tool does rely on an individual's (or few individuals') assessment of a clinical scenario. Due to the retrospective and somewhat subjective nature of reviews using this tool, published interrater agreement has been low.[19] However, this tool is widely used, accessible, and applicable to many different contexts, making it an appealing initial tool to use when analyzing cases. The SaferDx suite of tools is aimed primarily at identifying if a diagnostic error occurred; whereas causative factors leading to the error may be suggested in the course of completing the tool in a given case, the specific information generated may not be granular enough to guide and enable reflection and improvement.

The Diagnostic Error Evaluation and Research (DEER) Taxonomy is another tool used to evaluate diagnostic error events. Although the SaferDx tool involves adjudicating whether an error occurred, the DEER taxonomy tool is used to determine whereby deviations in the diagnostic process contributed to the error.[20] Although this tool also relies on individual assessment of a clinical scenario, interrater reliability of the DEER classification was moderate.[20]

Both the SaferDx and DEER taxonomy provide value by delineating and mapping if and whereby an error occurred; no current tool, however, describes why an error occurred. Truly understanding why deviations in the diagnostic process occurred is challenging and reflects the reality that diagnosis is a complex process that occurs in a specific context. Contextual features that are not captured in medical records but that significantly impact diagnostic reasoning include features of the work environment (eg, workload, distractions, interruptions, teamwork), patient factors (eg, language barriers, delirium, lack of trust in the health care system), and clinician factors (eg, fatigue, stress level).[21,22] Therefore, discussion with—and engagement of—clinicians in analyzing cases for improvement is crucial; involved clinicians are able to provide key contextual information that allows robust reflection and identification of both cognitive and systems factors that may be improved in future cases.

Another way to prevent errors is to recognize opportunities for improvement, even when an error did not occur. "Good catches" are cases with potential errors which did not occur. Recognizing and celebrating these events is a positive approach to both errors and patient safety. Review of potential errors allows a more proactive discussion about how to prevent future errors and identification of system fixes that can help. Clinicians are more likely to report positive findings which are likely why "good catches" are more frequently reported than "close calls."[23]

Retrospective case review is focused on learning from previous cases to prevent future errors. One such example of this is the medical peer review process whereby peer clinicians review cases to evaluate the care provided. Peer review is useful because the reviewers are fellow clinicians working in the same system and aware of local culture and barriers and have some protection from discoverability in litigation. Often the referrals are based on reporting systems or triggers mentioned previously, complaints or referrals from quality, risk management/legal, or other departments. The referral process itself leads to sampling issues because there are cases recognized for something that went wrong; further, there may be social determinants that may make a patient and/or family more or less likely to report a concern about a case or pursue legal action. Thus, analyzing and reflecting only on these cases may lead to conclusions and practice changes that may worsen disparities in the diagnostic process. Further, although being an important and relatively ubiquitous means by which cases are analyzed in a confidential manner, the peer-review process may be viewed by clinicians as punitive in nature. Cases addressed in peer review tend to be "high acuity, low frequency" events, and thus the process does not likely lead to consistent opportunities for reflection or improvement. Except for a (very) few instances, attributing a patient outcome to the actions or decisions of one clinician is not accurate, especially in a complex system with many interdependent parts like modern health care.[24]

Recommendations: How to Track Improvement

To make peer review a meaningful system, there should be 2 concurrent systems that operate synergistically. The first system is to recognize the error and the impact that error has on patients, families, and health care providers. The decisions and errors involved should be recognized and investigated to ensure such things do not happen again—a common refrain shared by patients and families affected by diagnostic and other medical errors.[25] Dedicated, formal, collaborative, and standard investigation into the events leading to the error along with the decisions made can provide further insight into how and the error occurred.[17] Identifying the specifics that made the error possible is imperative to preventing the same errors in the future. Similarly, identifying the impact of the error humanizes the issue for clinicians and administrators alike. Recognizing the error without reflection on the impact could make the process seem like an exercise or administrative task rather than a key opportunity for learning and improvement.

The second system should involve ongoing feedback to clinicians on decisions made. If clinicians are accustomed to receiving regular feedback, it removes the punitive nature of peer review because there is also ongoing positive and constructive feedback. Normalizing clinical feedback will help diminish the disciplinary nature of peer review and increase the acceptance of the feedback to make individual and systems changes. Moving from a "no news is good news" default system to a system where feedback about diagnostic decision-making and diagnostic outcomes is expected will help develop better calibrated clinicians who improve over time.[6,26] Calibration relates to a clinician's confidence in a decision relative to the accuracy of that decision, and better calibration—so that clinicians are neither too overconfident (and potentially dangerous) nor too underconfident (and prone to excessive testing)—is the goal of most modern diagnosis improvement programs.

Learning from Excellence

Seeking to improve diagnosis involves not only avoiding errors but also aiming for excellence; if we only seek to avoid diagnostic errors, we may develop a diagnostic process that is, safer but overly expensive, cumbersome, and replete with downstream harms. Fields outside of medicine that require high levels of human performance and relentless pursuit of improvement, such as professional sports, exemplify this process; athletes analyze games, and plays not only whereby success was not achieved but also when they excelled. Such analysis and learning from excellence also seek to engage clinicians in a different emotional context than cases of error alone, allowing best practices and "pearls" to be identified and disseminated to other clinicians. Said differently, just like cases in which diagnostic errors occurred may be analyzed to identify potential opportunities for improvement, cases of diagnostic excellence may similarly be analyzed for opportunities to improve other cases. Of course, finding cases in which diagnostic excellence occurred is even more challenging than identifying cases in which diagnostic errors occurred; however, it is likely that many of the reporting systems, case conferences, and even trigger tools could be adapted to seek excellence in addition to errors and adverse events.

How Does Diagnostic Improvement Actually Occur?

Once cases are identified and analyzed to identify opportunities for improvement, how does this improvement actually occur? Revisiting the stages of the learning process above, abstraction and planning for the future follow, and experience and reflection on it. This process of abstraction and future planning allow knowledge to be restructured and, if needed, knowledge gaps rectified. Clinicians' medical knowledge tends to be extensively organized in a process called encapsulation, and these highly structured, interdependent cognitive structures need to be continually revisited and refined to ensure they remain accessible, accurate, and up-to-date.[27]

Best Practices in Case Conferences

Another mechanism for retrospective review is the MMC in which clinicians and hospital administrators learn from individual and system errors. Although MMCs are held as educational conferences with the goal to improve patient care but by recognizing system errors, they are also great avenues for quality improvement. Often MMCs focus on pathophysiology and do not leave to actionable ideas to improve care and prevent future errors. Cases referred for MMC usually involve more serious harm which immediately skews the lens through which the case is reviewed. Alternatively, the MMCs that involve rare conditions or unique presentations may detract from the purpose of identifying the types and etiology of errors. Previous work to help improve MMCs has been to implement a systems-based approach to investigate and intervene on cases referred by clinicians and provide feedback on improvement efforts from previous cases to improve the process of reviewing and responding to adverse events.[28]

It is important during the reflection and evaluation of a case to keep in mind what the normal process should be. The concept of normalization of deviance describes whereby a defective operation of a system is recognized as normal and acceptable.[29] In other words, we become accustomed to system flaws as the norm and expectation which should not be the case. Acknowledging system deficiencies and other factors that may contribute to errors is imperative to continued growth. In addition, patients and clinicians are not accustomed to the occurrence of errors which may be personally and professionally jarring for everyone involved. Clinicians especially have a strong sense of denial related to errors which lead to further distrust. Clinician-driven specific and tangible feedback on clinical reasoning and errors can lead to more acceptance and lead to constructive clinical changes.[30]

As clinicians become more comfortable identifying systems issues, it is also vital to consider the impact of other outside factors on the individual cognitive process. The concept of situativity theory describes the perspective that knowledge and thinking, as well as learning, are situated in experience and context.[24] Another way to frame this is that it is impossible to separate actions from the environment. Clinical decisions are impacted by the environment along with social, cultural, and cognitive constraints.

A "cognitive autopsy" as described by Croskerry can allow for comprehensive consideration of the multitude of factors that lead to a certain decision.[31] It must be noted, however, that although it is important to consider the role that cognitive biases play in diagnostic errors, retrospective identification of cognitive bias is fraught with limitations and strategies aimed at improving diagnosis by decreasing cognitive bias has been generally ineffective. Evaluation of clinical cases should move beyond the 1-dimension of assigning individual fault and toward recognition of the multitude of factors that contributed to cognitive failures, the diagnostic error, and the ultimate outcome. One example is the modified fishbone diagram which involves the evaluation of factors such as communication, cognitive processing, organizational issues, and context among many others to evaluate the etiology of a diagnostic error.[32] Multiple other interventions have aimed to provide systematic opportunities for trainees to examine their own cases and learn from them, with excellent results and self-perceived improvements in reasoning by those involved.[2,33] Another important project involved trainee reflection on patients they treated over a specific time frame. The learners were given the opportunity to review the patients in the medical record and then report back their thoughts; this activity was viewed favorably by residents.

Providing feedback to clinicians on errors is a sensitive but imperative step in the improvement process. Due to fragmentation and efficiency-related silos created in medicine, clinicians are often not aware of the outcomes of their decisions. Iterative feedback on the outcomes of clinical decisions allows for calibration and offers the opportunity for learning and thus improvement.[34]

Reflection on Action in Diagnosis

Although there has been much focus in research, quality improvement, and education innovations on developing reliable and consistent methods to reflect on cases to improve future decision-making, methods to enable reflection in action are also important. Such methods are aimed at improving decision-making, avoiding common pitfalls, and avoiding diagnostic errors in real-time. Although many such potential methods have been suggested, the evidence regarding effectiveness is, in many cases, lacking.[35] There was initial enthusiasm for strategies to identify and avoid cognitive biases during diagnostic reasoning, as cognitive biases and other flaws in decision-making do play a role in diagnostic errors. However, such strategies, often called metacognition, have generally not been shown to be effective at improving diagnostic outcomes.[35] This limitation is likely because although flaws in the underlying cognitive processes used to make decisions may contribute to diagnostic errors, gaps in context-specific knowledge contribute substantially to diagnostic errors.

Checklists are commonly used during other processes in medicine (and other fields) to ensure standard work and avoid adverse events; their use has been suggested as a means to improve diagnostic performance.[36,37] Checklists aimed at improving diagnosis may be general (ie, aimed at ensuring that steps in the diagnostic process are followed and common pitfalls avoided) or specific (ie, aimed at avoiding pitfalls and pursuing a complete differential diagnosis for a given concern). Diagnostic timeouts have also been suggested as a means to improve diagnostic performance, but there remain significant questions about which cases will benefit from a diagnostic timeout.[38] This question is especially important given the fact that studies of diagnostic accuracy have generally not shown that more time spent leads to better diagnostic performance.[39]

One of the most promising strategies to improve diagnostic performance in real-time is through the use of structured reflection; this process prompts the clinician to apply context-specific knowledge to evaluate and weigh clinical information that either supports or refutes an item on a differential diagnosis for a given case.[40] This structured reflection process encourages clinicians to consider each item on the differential diagnosis in turn and consider what pieces of information argue for or against that item, as well as what clinical features would be expected but are missing in a given case. It must be noted, however, that studies of structured reflection have been limited to research and educational settings, and some adaptations have not led to improvements in diagnostic performance. However, the structured reflection method seems to hold significant promise as a context-specific and content-specific strategy to improve diagnosis.

Future Directions

Reflection—either in action or on action—requires that an individual be presented with outcomes of their decisions, often defined as feedback. Thus, there is an inextricable link between reflection and feedback. One of the first questions that relate to enabling reflective practice in diagnosis is, "What do we give feedback about to enable effective reflection?" Most clinical encounters in modern health care include a vast amount of data, complex reasoning, and variable time courses that make answering this question quite difficult. Since diagnosis can be viewed as both process and outcome, feedback must occur about both the diagnostic process and diagnostic outcomes. Further, although diagnostic processes and diagnostic outcomes are linked, this relationship is neither predestined nor linear; good processes do not always lead to good outcomes, whereas suboptimal outcomes do not always mean a flawed process. In addition, it is likely quite important to learn from both being wrong (diagnostic errors) and from being right (diagnostic excellence). Intentional and consistent reflection on cases provides an opportunity to review what has been conducted before and also reinforces decisions that were made. Reflection and discussion in a supportive environment can help manage cognitive and diagnostic uncertainty.[41]

SUMMARY

Given the complexities of these realities, the task of implementing methods to enable feedback and reflection about diagnostic decision-making and performance may seem daunting; however, important steps have been made in recent years that have started to lay the evidence base for high-quality, effective, and sustainable reflective diagnostic practice to occur.

CLINICS CARE POINTS

- Reflection on action: a person looks back on a decision or event and consider how the decision, its underlying processes and context impacted an outcome.
- Reflection in action: a person is able to consider a decision, its underlying processes and context in near-real time to modify a decision and outcomes.
- Incident reporting and triggered tools in the electronic health record can be useful in error recognition.
- Learning from diagnostic reflection must include both feedback regarding errors along with recognition of diagnostic excellence.

DISCLOSURE

The authors have nothing to disclose.

REFERENCES

1. Sandars J. The use of reflection in medical education: AMEE Guide No. 44. Med Teach 2009;31(8):685–95.
2. Lane KP, Chia C, Lessing JN, et al. Improving resident feedback on diagnostic reasoning after handovers: the LOOP project. J Hosp Med 2019;14(10):E1–625.
3. Institute of Medicine Committee on Quality of Health Care in A. In: Kohn LT, Corrigan JM, Donaldson MS, editors. To err is human: building a safer health system. National Academies Press (US) Copyright 2000 by the National Academy of Sciences. All rights reserved; 2000.

4. Berner ES, Graber ML. Overconfidence as a cause of diagnostic error in medicine. Am J Med 2008;121(5 Suppl):S2–23.
5. Olson A, Rencic J, Cosby K, et al. Competencies for improving diagnosis: an interprofessional framework for education and training in health care. Diagnosis (Berl) 2019;6(4):335–41.
6. Fernandez Branson C, Williams M, Chan TM, et al. Improving diagnostic performance through feedback: the diagnosis learning cycle. BMJ Qual Saf 2021. https://doi.org/10.1136/bmjqs-2020-012456.
7. Newman-Toker DE. A unified conceptual model for diagnostic errors: underdiagnosis, overdiagnosis, and misdiagnosis. Diagnosis (Berl) 2014;1(1):43–8.
8. Gleason KT, Peterson S, Kasda E, et al. Capturing diagnostic errors in incident reporting systems: value of a specific "DX Tile" for diagnosis-related concerns. Diagnosis (Berl) 2018;5(4):249–51.
9. Elder NC, Graham D, Brandt E, et al. Barriers and motivators for making error reports from family medicine offices: a report from the American Academy of Family Physicians National Research Network (AAFP NRN). J Am Board Fam Med 2007;20(2):115–23.
10. King ES, Moyer DV, Couturie MJ, et al. Getting doctors to report medical errors: project DISCLOSE. Jt Comm J Qual Patient Saf 2006;32(7):382–92.
11. Marshall TL, Ipsaro AJ, Le M, et al. Increasing physician reporting of diagnostic learning opportunities. Pediatrics (Evanston) 2021;147(1):e20192400.
12. Murphy DR, Meyer AN, Sittig DF, et al. Application of electronic trigger tools to identify targets for improving diagnostic safety. BMJ Qual Saf 2019;28(2):151–9.
13. Landrigan CP, Stockwell D, Toomey SL, et al. Performance of the global assessment of pediatric patient safety (GAPPS) tool. Pediatrics 2016;137(6):e20154076.
14. Murphy DR, Meyer AND, Vaghani V, et al. Development and validation of trigger algorithms to identify delays in diagnostic evaluation of gastroenterological cancer. Clin Gastroenterol Hepatol 2018;16(1):90–8.
15. Vaghani V, Wei L, Mushtaq U, et al. Validation of an electronic trigger to measure missed diagnosis of stroke in emergency departments. J Am Med Inform Assoc 2021. https://doi.org/10.1093/jamia/ocab121.
16. Al-Mutairi A, Meyer AND, Thomas EJ, et al. Accuracy of the safer dx instrument to identify diagnostic errors in primary care. J Gen Intern Med 2016;31(6):602–8.
17. Singh H, Khanna A, Spitzmueller C, et al. Recommendations for using the revised safer Dx Instrument to help measure and improve diagnostic safety. Diagnosis (Berlin, Germany) 2019;6(4):315–23.
18. Davalos MC, Samuels K, Meyer AND, et al. Finding diagnostic errors in children admitted to the PICU. Pediatr Crit Care Med 2017;18(3):265–71.
19. Zwaan L, de Bruijne M, Wagner C, et al. Patient record review of the incidence, consequences, and causes of diagnostic adverse events. Arch Intern Med 2010;170(12):1015–21.
20. Schiff GD, Hasan O, Kim S, et al. Diagnostic error in medicine: analysis of 583 physician-reported errors. Arch Intern Med 2009;169(20):1881–7.
21. Olson APJ, Durning SJ, Fernandez Branson C, et al. Teamwork in clinical reasoning - cooperative or parallel play? Diagnosis (Berl) 2020;7(3):307–12.
22. Konopasky A, Artino AR, Battista A, et al. Understanding context specificity: the effect of contextual factors on clinical reasoning. Diagnosis (Berl) 2020;7(3):257–64.
23. Mick JM, Wood GL, Massey RL. The good catch pilot program: increasing potential error reporting. J Nurs Adm 2007;37(11):499–503.

24. Durning SJ, Artino AR. Situativity theory: a perspective on how participants and the environment can interact: AMEE Guide no. 52. Med Teach 2011;33(3): 188–99.
25. Giardina TD, Korukonda S, Shahid U, et al. Use of patient complaints to identify diagnosis-related safety concerns: a mixed-method evaluation. BMJ Qual Saf 2021. https://doi.org/10.1136/bmjqs-2020-011593.
26. Meyer AND, Singh H. The path to diagnostic excellence includes feedback to calibrate how clinicians think. JAMA 2019;321(8):737–8.
27. Schmidt H, Boshuizen H. On acquiring expertise in medicine. Educ Psychol Rev 1993;5(3):205–21.
28. Cifra CL, Bembea MM, Fackler JC, et al. Transforming the morbidity and mortality conference to promote safety and quality in a PICU. Pediatr Crit Care Med 2016; 17(1):58–66.
29. Vaughan D. The challenger launch decision: risky technology, culture, and deviance at NASA. Chicago (IL): University of Chicago Press; 1996.
30. Wu AW, Folkman S, McPhee SJ, et al. How house officers cope with their mistakes. West J Med 1993;159(5):565–9.
31. Croskerry P. Diagnostic failure: a cognitive and affective approach. In: Henriksen K, Battles JB, Marks ES, et al, editors. Advances in Patient Safety: From Research to Implementation (Volume 2: Concepts and Methodology). Rockville (MD): Agency for Healthcare Research and Quality (US); 2005.
32. Reilly JB, Myers JS, Salvador D, et al. Use of a novel, modified fishbone diagram to analyze diagnostic errors. Diagnosis (Berl) 2014;1(2):167–71.
33. Ogdie AR, Reilly JB, Pang WG, et al. Seen through their eyes: residents' reflections on the cognitive and contextual components of diagnostic errors in medicine. Acad Med 2012;87(10):1361–7.
34. Croskerry P. The feedback sanction. Acad Emerg Med 2000;7(11):1232–8.
35. Norman GR, Monteiro SD, Sherbino J, et al. The causes of errors in clinical reasoning: cognitive biases, knowledge deficits, and dual process thinking. Acad Med 2017;92(1):23–30.
36. Ely JW, Graber ML, Croskerry P. Checklists to reduce diagnostic errors. Acad Med 2011;86(3):307–13.
37. Ely JW, Graber MA. Checklists to prevent diagnostic errors: a pilot randomized controlled trial. Diagnosis (Berl) 2015;2(3):163–9.
38. Trowbridge RL. Twelve tips for teaching avoidance of diagnostic errors. Med Teach 2008;30(5):496–500.
39. Staal J, Alsma J, Mamede S, et al. The relationship between time to diagnose and diagnostic accuracy among internal medicine residents: a randomized experiment. BMC Med Educ 2021;21(1):227.
40. Mamede S, Goeijenbier M, Schuit SCE, et al. Specific disease knowledge as predictor of susceptibility to availability bias in diagnostic reasoning: a randomized controlled experiment. J Gen Intern Med 2021;36(3):640–6.
41. Sommers LS, Morgan L, Johnson L, et al. Practice inquiry: clinical uncertainty as a focus for small-group learning and practice improvement. J Gen Intern Med 2007;22(2):246–52.

Promoting Critical Thinking in Your Intensive Care Unit Team

Jeremy B. Richards, MD, MA*, Richard M. Schwartzstein, MD

KEYWORDS

- Critical thinking • Clinical reasoning • Clinical decision making • Metacognition
- Cognitive biases • Critical care • Medical education

KEY POINTS

- Critical thinking is defined as efficiently and effectively analyzing or evaluating medical information to make decisions that are precise, logical, accurate, and appropriate.
- The intensive care unit is a dynamic and challenging environment where volume and complexity of data increases the risk of cognitive errors, morbidity, and mortality.
- Identifying and defining cognitive biases is an important strategy to decrease the risk of cognitive error.
- Concept or mechanism maps can be used to diagnose disorganized thinking and to reinforce inductive reasoning and key connections and concepts in clinical practice.
- Active teaching strategies such as think-pair-share and using "how" and "why" questions can support and promote critical thinking skills in medical learners and ICU team members.

INTRODUCTION

The intensive care unit (ICU) is a challenging and dynamic clinical environment where the potential for cognitive and clinical errors is significant. As many as 40,500 ICU patients in the United States may die with misdiagnoses each year,[1] due to faulty clinical reasoning resulting in diagnostic errors.[2] Patients may experience up to 1.7 errors per day in the ICU,[3] and almost every critically ill ICU patient will experience a potentially life-threatening error during their clinical course.[4] Diagnostic errors, which typically represent thinking or cognitive mistakes, have been estimated to contribute to 5% to 10% of adverse events and contribute to death, permanent disability, or prolonged hospital length of stay.[5] Human failure is the main cause of diagnostic errors resulting in adverse events,[6] although capacity strain and distractions in the ICU can increase

Division of Pulmonary, Critical Care, and Sleep Medicine, Beth Israel Deaconess Medical Center, 330, Brookline Avenue, KS-B23, Boston, MA 02215, USA
* Corresponding author.
E-mail address: jbrichar@bidmc.harvard.edu
Twitter: @jbricha1 (J.B.R.)

Crit Care Clin 38 (2022) 113–127
https://doi.org/10.1016/j.ccc.2021.08.002
0749-0704/22/© 2021 Elsevier Inc. All rights reserved.

the risk of adverse patient outcomes, including increased morbidity and mortality.[7–9] In this context, the frequency of cognitive and clinical errors in the ICU represents an opportunity for improved care by promoting and optimizing clinical reasoning and critical thinking skills in ICU teams.

At face value, teaching critical thinking skills to medical trainees seems desirable; however, understanding what constitutes "critical thinking" is important for clinicians and educators, to ensure that educational interventions and efforts achieve the desired goals. In the practice of medicine, critical thinking can be conceptualized differently depending on context and perspective. Specifically, while biomedical critical thinking is the dominant conception of critical thinking in medical practice, humanist and social justice–oriented critical thinking skills have also been described.[10] Humanist conceptions of critical thinking are directed toward social good and intimately related to interpersonal interactions and relationships and compliment biomedical critical thinking by emphasizing psychosocial and relational aspects of clinical practice.[10] Social justice–oriented critical thinking focuses on identifying and addressing assumptions and biases and requires understanding of the social systems in which health care activities take place.[10] While we will focus on biomedical critical thinking skills, awareness of the different conceptions and manifestations of such skills indicates that a consensus definition of "critical thinking" may not be easily obtainable.

Defining the Concept of "Critical Thinking"

With regard to biomedical critical thinking, authors and experts have provided varying definitions of critical thinking, emphasizing attributes such as "intellectual discipline" and behaviors such as "conceptualizing, applying, analyzing, synthesizing, and/or evaluating" in an effort to describe the cognitive processes of critical thinking skills.[11,12] Despite the lack of a consensus definition,[10,13] with variable definitions of critical thinking in the literature,[14] the most pertinent description for the practice of medicine was developed in an expert consensus conference in 2011:

"[C]ritical thinking in the clinical context [is] the application of higher cognitive skills (eg, conceptualization, analysis, evaluation) to information (gathered from medical history, records, physical exam, or diagnostic investigation) in a way that leads to action that is, precise, consistent, logical, and appropriate."[15]

While some consider critical thinking skills to be a disposition or state, most medical educators consider critical thinking to be a process or ability and, therefore, teachable.[16] Milestones of critical thinking in medical education and practice have been described, based on consensus agreement of medical educators, informed by developmental stage theories.[17] These proposed milestones of critical thinking are specific to health care education and describe different levels of metacognition, attitudes, and skills (**Table 1**). "Best strategies" to teach and promote critical thinking abilities in medical learners, however, have not been rigorously described or assessed in the literature. In this context, we review several educational approaches to promote critical thinking and related cognitive skills in medical learners in the ICU.

Promoting Critical Thinking for Learners

Critical thinking skills encompass related attributes and abilities such as curiosity, inquisitiveness, and metacognition (the process of thinking about one's thinking). As such, promoting critical thinking skills necessarily involves fostering and supporting these related attributes. The educational strategies described here variably emphasize different aspects of critical thinking, with the goal of holistically developing the breadth

Table 1
Milestones of critical thinking in health care education, with levels of metacognition, attitudes, and skills

Stage of Critical Thinking	Metacognition	Attitudes	Skills
Stage 1: unreflective thinker	Does not demonstrate the ability to examine their own actions and cognitive processes	Lack of flexibility, fixation on working beliefs, inability to accept ambiguity or adapt to new knowledge	Single approach to gathering and processing information (eg, rote memorization)
Stage 2: beginning critical thinker	Nascent awareness of different thinking strategies, preliminary recognition of cognitive differences in others	Receptive to feedback about their thinking, but rarely asks for or seeks out feedback	Intermittent use of different cognitive strategies, recognition of the importance of foundational principles but infrequently applies them in clinical reasoning
Stage 3: practicing critical thinker	Familiarity with metacognitive theories and attempts to apply them in their own clinical reasoning	Acknowledges uncertainties, open to challenges about their thinking and decision making, and accepts new reasoning approaches	Acknowledges and uses different strategies to solve clinical problems, and uses established principles to guide decisions
Stage 4: advanced critical thinker	Uses several different approaches to thinking, and can identify ways in which others' thinking is distinct from their own	Actively seeks out and accepts feedback about their own thinking	Pivots between intuitive and analytical skills to solve problems, and adjusts thinking strategies as needed based on context and to avoid cognitive biases
Stage 5: accomplished critical thinker	Uses theories of metacognition to habitually monitor, revise, and rethink approaches for continual improvement of cognitive strategies	Actively works to improve their own and others' thinking strategies, and openly acknowledges assumptions, uncertainty, and biases	Models critical thinking skills to others, including when and how to transition from pattern recognition to analytical reasoning, and can create new knowledge and understanding through inductive reasoning

Adapted from Papp KK, Huang GC, Lauzon Clabo LM, et al. Milestones of critical thinking: a developmental model for medicine and nursing. Acad Med J Assoc Am Med Coll. 2014;89(5):715-720. https://doi.org/10.1097/ACM.0000000000000220; with permission.

of cognitive abilities that result in effective, logical, analytical, and appropriate clinical decision-making.

Identify and Define Cognitive Biases

There are numerous cognitive biases or heuristics (ie, mental shortcuts) that affect how we think and make decisions. Cognitive biases leverage pattern recognition, allowing one to make a rapid and relatively effortless conclusion in response to a set of observations. Pattern recognition, referred to as "System 1" processing in the dual process model of clinical reasoning, is contrasted by more cognitively effortful, analytical, and systematic processing referred to as "System 2" processing.[18] In the ICU, pattern recognition has a role in helping health care providers process the large volume of information to which they are exposed, but it is more prone to systematic errors and cognitive biasing than System 2 reasoning.

The simple act of discussing these different modes of reasoning, System 1 versus System 2 reasoning, may encourage ICU team members to engage in metacognition, a core component of effective critical thinking. As noted previously, metacognition is defined as "thinking about your thinking" — it is the process of being aware of how one is approaching and thinking through a problem, as well as being cognizant of how much effort and focus one is dedicating to the topic or problem at hand.[19] Identifying, defining, and describing System 1 and System 2 modes of reasoning to ICU team members may encourage them to be more cognizant of their own thought patterns and processes while caring for patients in the ICU.[2,20]

In addition to identifying, defining, and describing the dual process theory of cognition and metacognition, naming, describing, and contextualizing specific cognitive biases will both increase awareness of these biases and their effects on critical thinking, as well as help team members identify an instance of falling victim to these errors. Furthermore, reasoning from basic physiologic and pathologic principles of disease to explain clinical findings (inductive reasoning),[21] rather than jumping quickly to a disease-centric differential diagnosis (hypothetico-deductive reasoning),[22] may diminish the risk of cognitive mistakes. Given that learners often are more prone to System 1 thinking because of their reliance on illness scripts and, consequently, may be at increased risk of falling victim to cognitive biases and errors in clinical reasoning, we will describe two of the most common cognitive biases in the following sections.

Anchoring bias

Anchoring bias is a powerful cognitive bias that is defined as making a diagnosis early in a patient's presentation based on a limited set of clinical data and subsequently failing to modify the initial diagnosis despite newer (and potentially contradictory) information.[2] Anchoring bias commonly manifests in clinical practice and is related to confirmation bias, another common cognitive bias. Confirmation bias is defined as the tendency to look for confirming evidence to support a diagnosis, as opposed to looking for contradictory evidence to refute the initial diagnosis.[2] Sometimes referred to as "seizing and freezing," anchoring bias reflects the predilection to settle on a diagnosis (or decision) after which one stops putting in cognitive effort to continue to analyze subsequent clinical information.

Diagnostic errors occurred in up to 77% of case scenarios because of anchoring bias in a recent systematic review, demonstrating the prevalence and importance of this cognitive bias on medical decision-making.[23] Anchoring bias can significantly influence both patient and physician perceptions of diagnostic likelihood in different clinical scenarios. Specifically, presenting irrelevant numeric anchors to patients and physicians can significantly alter their estimations of the likelihood of specific diagnoses causing a patient's presenting signs and symptoms.[24] Discussing anchoring bias with ICU team members can have an unmasking effect, and identifying instances of anchoring bias in the context of actual clinical cases may serve to decrease the frequency of and mitigate against the detrimental effects of anchoring.[25]

System-based changes may also help to decrease the propensity to fall victim to anchoring bias, including emphasizing structured diagnostic assessments and computer-based decision-support tools.[26,27] However, the efficacy of such system-based tools is inevitably influenced by the individual health care provider using the tools, such that the teaching and promotion of individual critical thinking skills is necessary to optimize the efficacy of decision-support tools.

Availability bias

Availability bias can manifest differently depending on context. One manifestation of availability bias is that a diagnosis is thought to be more likely if it easily comes to mind in a clinical scenario. Conversely, availability bias can also manifest by assuming that a diagnosis is unlikely because it either did not occur to the health care provider early in the encounter or because the health care provider has infrequently seen that diagnosis cause the patient's presenting signs or symptoms.

As an example, if a health care provider in the ICU is assessing a patient with chest pain, hypotension, and shortness of breath and had recently cared for three patients with submassive pulmonary emboli who presented with similar symptoms, the provider is prone to overestimate the likelihood that the current patient has a pulmonary embolism. Conversely, if a provider has never seen a case of thrombotic thrombocytopenia purpura, that diagnosis may not readily come to mind and may be discounted as being unlikely, even if a patient presents with the pentad of microangiopathic hemolytic anemia, thrombocytopenia, fever, neurologic symptoms, and uremia.

Availability is a powerful cognitive bias and has been demonstrated to significantly affect clinical reasoning in simulated clinical reasoning scenarios. Specifically, in one study in which internal medicine residents were asked to provide diagnoses in response to a series of clinical vignettes, introducing availability bias by providing vignettes similar to those they had already seen but with different diagnoses, diagnostic accuracy was significantly negatively impacted.[28] Availability bias can be mitigated, however, by using an analytical reasoning approach for assessing case scenarios (**Box 1**).[28]

Identifying availability bias is the first step in combatting its effects on critical thinking and clinical reasoning; naming and defining this cognitive bias is an important means of promoting critical thinking in ICU teams. Modeling the use of analytical

---

Box 1
Strategies for decreasing the risk of committing availability bias

Analytical reasoning strategy to decrease the risk of availability bias:
1. Read the case
2. Write prior diagnosis
3. List pertinent positives
4. List pertinent negatives
5. List expected, but absent, pertinent positives

Data from Mamede S, van Gog T, van den Berge K, et al. Effect of availability bias and reflective reasoning on diagnostic accuracy among internal medicine residents. JAMA. 2010;304(11):1198-1203. https://doi.org/10.1001/jama.2010.1276.

reasoning approaches to mitigate availability bias will encourage ICU team members to approach clinical scenarios systematically, thereby decreasing the risk of falling victim to this cognitive error.

Debiasing strategies

Debiasing strategies may help health care providers avoid common cognitive biases. Awareness of and engagement in metacognition is thought to be an important strategy for decreasing the frequency and severity of committing cognitive biases, although it should be acknowledged that this is an effortful process.[29] Explicitly acknowledging uncertainty is another strategy for decreasing the risk of anchoring on a diagnosis or prematurely closing one's consideration of alternative diagnoses.[30] Using Bayesian reasoning to diagnostic evaluations and decision-making is another strategy to quantify clinical reasoning and to minimize the effects of intuition, assumptions, or impressions on the diagnostic reasoning process.[31]

The effectiveness of debiasing strategies ultimately, and understandably, is influenced by the effort one puts into the strategies. A superficial approach to debiasing strategies will result in minimal gains and will not effectively decrease the risk of falling victim to cognitive biases or committing diagnostic errors. As such, support of and feedback regarding the use of debiasing strategies is an important component of the ultimate efficacy of these strategies on clinical reasoning and critical thinking skills.[32]

Create a Clinical Learning Environment Conducive to Critical Thinking

A supportive, safe, and conducive clinical learning environment is critical for promoting and supporting medical learners' critical thinking skills. Attending physicians can develop a conducive learning environment by explicitly modeling effective clinical reasoning skills (ie, by explaining the thought process and metacognition at play), embracing uncertainty, using active teaching techniques, and promoting inductive as opposed to deductive clinical reasoning.[30] These strategies are discussed in detail in the following sections.

Promoting a learner environment that emphasizes "psychological safety" is an important component of developing a clinical learning environment that fosters and promotes learners' critical thinking skills.[33] The norms, values, expectations, and behaviors exhibited by attending physicians directly affects the explicit and hidden curricula and become a part of the culture of practice in the ICU. Attendings who dismiss, humiliate, shame, or embarrass learners contribute to an ineffective learning environment and inhibit learners' ability to develop clinical reasoning and critical thinking skills.[34] Understanding the role of psychological safety in medical education and allowing learners to describe their clinical reasoning processes while providing supportive and constructive feedback is a key leadership skill for helping learners develop and refine their critical thinking abilities.[35,36]

Cognitive Timeouts

Similar to the concept of a procedural "timeout," a cognitive timeout is an opportunity to pause and reflect on a patient's diagnosis or clinical circumstances by reviewing the available evidence and thought processes that led to the working diagnosis.[37] Cognitive timeouts (or "diagnostic pauses") have been evaluated in the outpatient setting and have demonstrated changes in both diagnostic assessments as well as clinical management among primary care providers in a manner that was both feasible and acceptable.[38] While cognitive timeouts have not been formally studied in the ICU setting, the positive results in other clinical settings suggest that the process of pausing and reflecting on a diagnosis may be similarly beneficial for ICU providers.[39]

Awareness of cognitive biases is an essential component of performing an effective cognitive timeout; to decrease the risk of merely reviewing the available data and getting the same result, one must reframe the clinical scenario to truly question the current diagnosis. Reframing the initial approach to the patient and their diagnosis enables the physician to truly take a new perspective on the case, to consider alternative hypotheses, and to challenge the prior assessment. Such reframing will allow the practitioner to avoid repeating cognitive biases and/or diagnostic errors that resulted in the initial, established diagnosis.

Cognitive timeouts may be particularly beneficial for patients who are not improving with treatments that, in theory, should have addressed the patient's problem because the presence of diagnostic error in critically ill patients frequently accounts for poor outcomes. Obtaining broad input from team members during a cognitive time out can leverage the power of teamwork by ensuring that different perspectives from providers of different disciplines (eg, nursing, pharmacy, respiratory therapy, and so forth) and input from learners and providers at different levels of training are considered. Numerous studies have demonstrated improved diagnostic accuracy attributable to working in teams as opposed to working individually to solve medical problems, and the role of the team can be leveraged to optimize the impact of cognitive timeouts in the ICU.[40–42] Cognitive timeouts cannot be performed every day on every patient, but they may be a useful exercise for select patients, and a cognitive timeout provides an opportunity to explicitly model and practice the analytical, systematic approach of System 2 reasoning.[18]

Active Teaching Strategies

By explicitly engaging team members in critical thinking, one can promote analytical reasoning skills in the ICU team. Leveraging active teaching and learning techniques is a powerful and evidence-based means of promoting core elements of critical thinking, such as evaluation of data, analytical reasoning skills, and developing cogent and rational conclusions. There are a variety of evidence-based active teaching strategies that can be used in both formal teaching sessions as well as in the clinical setting to support the development of critical thinking skills.

Think-pair-share

Think-pair-share was initially described over 40 years ago by Lyman and McTiGHE.[43] Think-pair-share is a simple educational intervention that can be deployed in a variety of settings, from formal classroom or conference room–based venues to the clinical environment. This strategy has been incorporated into various educational interventions, from case-based collaborative learning to flipped classroom teaching.[44,45] Think-pair-share has been extensively evaluated over the past 40 years and has consistently demonstrated improved knowledge and behavioral outcomes and improved performance in medical learners in both the classroom and clinical setting.

Think-pair-share may be deployed in the ICU in formal teaching settings (eg, a pre-rounds or postrounds teaching session) and/or as part of work rounds (eg, a brief pause on rounds for a think-pair-share activity). In the clinical setting, during breaks in rounds, such as when the attending has to answer a page, a think-pair-share exercise could be used to engage team members to brainstorm diagnostic impressions on challenging patients or develop clinical hypotheses to explain a patient's signs of symptoms.

The data supporting this approach as an effective, engaging educational intervention in medical education are substantive and span several decades, although the bulk of the evidence is in the classroom-based setting.[46,47] Think-pair-share can be variably deployed depending on context and circumstances. Groups of two to four team members can be used for the "pair" portion of the exercise, and the "share" component can be flexible with one, two, or all "pairs" reporting out after considering a discussion question or prompt. The flexibility of think-pair-share allows for it to be adapted to the learners, the setting, and the educational and clinical needs in the moment. The foundation of this technique in peer learning contributes to its ability to engage the student and/or resident and to its effectiveness.

"How" and "why" questions

Strategic and well-phrased questions can engage learners and team members' critical thinking skills in the ICU. Specifically, instead of prioritizing fact-based "what" questions, using inquiries that ask "why" and "how" as antecedents can encourage team members to leverage analytical, critical thinking skills, as opposed to accessing content knowledge via closed-ended responses.[48] Closed-ended questions that start with "what" can be perceived as threatening, as the implication from "what"-based questions is that there is a single correct answer. Furthermore, "what"-based questions can usually be answered through a quick internet search and do not leverage higher order critical thinking skills nor assess understanding of pathophysiological principles that manifest as symptoms, signs, and laboratory abnormalities and permit the learner to truly ascend the Bloom's taxonomy of educational objectives.[48]

In contrast, questions that begin with "how" or "why" invite a learner or team member to explain their reasoning in a more open-ended manner and promote discussion and critical thinking skills in the clinical setting. Coupling "how" and "why" questions with well-described clinical teaching frameworks such as the One Minute Preceptor[49] and summarize, narrow, analyze, probe, plan, and self-directed teaching (SNAPPS)[50] can further support and promote critical thinking skills in medical learners and ICU team members. With these questions, the teacher can quickly assess gaps in knowledge and understanding, the ability of the learner to apply information to solve problems, and their aptitude to evaluate novel situations.

Reflective writing

Reflective writing is an effective strategy for promoting metacognition and for reflecting on clinical reasoning and critical thinking skills.[35] Reflective writing exercises can occur in the context of clinical practice (eg, developing thoughtful notes, particularly in articulating one's "impression and plans," that make one's reasoning explicit), or reflective writing can be a separate activity, removed from clinical work. Reflective writing, especially when focused on errors or mishaps in clinical care, can be effortful, and protected time to engage in reflective writing exercises can increase the effectiveness and perceived value of this activity. Furthermore, ICU team members and learners are unlikely to be familiar with reflective writing outside of the context of clinical documentation, such that modeling, guidance, and support will likely be necessary for the exercise to be beneficial. Reflective writing has been shown to help internal medicine residents identify and describe their own experiences with diagnostic errors and cognitive biases,[51] which directly links to critical thinking skills.

Concept or Mechanism Maps

Concept maps are graphic representations of one's knowledge or understanding about a topic or concept. As described by Novak and Gowin, classic concept maps are organized in a top-down hierarchical manner, with a primary concept positioned at the top of the map and supporting propositions or concepts arranged underneath the primary concept, connected by arrows and linking words (**Fig. 1**).[52] Mechanism

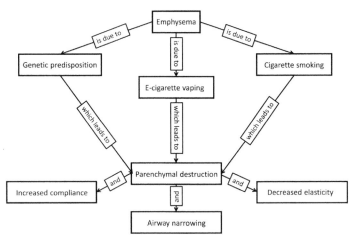

Fig. 1. Example of a concept map, with a hierarchical organization and use of connecting words between nodes.

maps are a more organic, less hierarchical variation of classic concept maps, which may better represent the complex interconnections of medical concepts (**Fig. 2**).[53] The effort of developing mechanism maps leverages key components of critical thinking, including analytical reasoning (How do these different concepts fit together?),[54] metacognition (How am I thinking about this problem?),[55] and mechanistic reasoning (Why does this sign or symptom occur in this disease process?),[56] which underlies the ability to apply an inductive process to solve the problem.

The impact of mechanism maps in medical education have primarily been assessed in the preclinical, classroom-based setting, and have been shown to enhance learners self-perceived reasoning skills, attitudes toward teamwork, and final examination performance, as compared to standard teaching practices.[53,57,58] While the bulk of the data regarding mechanism maps focus on classroom-based learning, the benefits of using mechanism maps can be extrapolated from the preclinical setting and applied to clinical learners, including in the ICU.

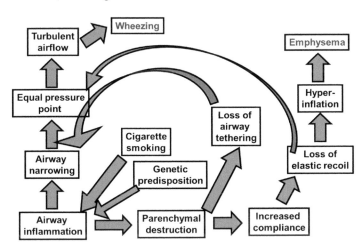

Fig. 2. Example of a mechanism map, with an organic, interconnected organization and implied connections between nodes.

Specifically, mechanism maps can be a powerful tool for teaching and can be used both in formal teaching sessions as well as in the context of clinical care. With regard to formal teaching sessions, prerounds or postrounds teaching sessions can focus on collaboratively developing a mechanism map about a clinical topic with learners. The educator can write out a discrete set of topics on a whiteboard, either clinical signs or symptoms and/or pathophysiologic mechanisms, and the teaching session can focus on identifying and developing the interconnections between these topics (**Fig. 3**). At the end of the teaching session, the educator and/or learners can take a picture of the whiteboard to preserve the collaboratively developed mechanism map for subsequent review.

During work rounds, a focused mechanism map, limited to one part of the patient's problem, for example, hypotension or hypoxemia, can assist with the analytical reasoning needed for direct patient care in the moment and can serve to reinforce how a critically ill patient's myriad and seemingly disparate issues can be linked together. If a learner is struggling to make connections between pathophysiologic mechanisms and clinical manifestations of a disease process, graphically demonstrating the mechanistic linkages on a piece of paper or whiteboard can provide visual scaffold for the concepts being discussed. Furthermore, developing a quick mechanism map to reinforce key points generates a durable resource that the learner can review after rounds.

While mechanism maps can be used for teaching and reinforcing key concepts and connections, they can also be used for assessment. Formal assessment practices for concept or mechanism maps have not been well described in the literature, but mechanism maps may be valuable in performing qualitative assessments of learners' disorganized thinking about a problem, topic, or concept.[59,60] Scoring systems for concept or mechanism maps vary significantly, and it is not clear that one assessment strategy is superior to another, such that holistic and qualitative assessments of learners' or team members' maps may be the optimal assessment approach at this time.

There are a variety of strategies for developing mechanism maps in formal teaching settings or at the bedside. Specifically, mechanism maps can be developed spontaneously in response to a relevant concept or topic that comes up during a teaching session or on rounds. This method of developing mechanism maps is useful for modeling critical thinking in real time but may be less preferable than using a preplanned map for linking learning to prior knowledge for the student or resident. Spontaneous maps are more prone to error and/or incomplete interconnections between

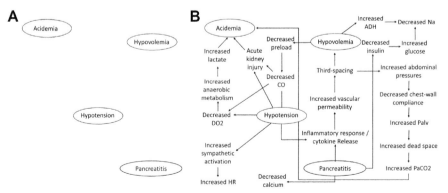

Fig. 3. Example of the beginning of a mechanism map in which the educator lists select nodes (*A*), and a "completed" mechanism map in which the learners connected the nodes with clinical and pathophysiologic mechanisms (*B*).

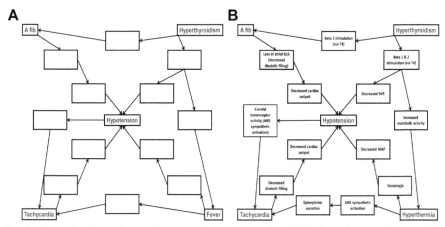

Fig. 4. Example of an "incomplete" mechanism map in which the educator has filled in some nodes and designated interconnections (*A*), and a "completed" mechanism map in which the learners have filled in the empty nodes (*B*).

nodes. A mechanism map constructed in advance of a teaching session can serve as a guide or "roadmap" for the map that is developed on the whiteboard with learners.

A variation on developing mechanism maps with or for learners is to have learners complete so-called "incomplete" mechanism maps. Specifically, the educator can provide both a discrete set of topics or concepts, as well as a series of blank nodes with prespecified interconnections (**Fig. 4**). Learners then can fill in the blanks in a rational and logical manner that links the prefilled nodes without having to concomitantly focus on identifying and defining interconnections between nodes. This method of filling in "incomplete" mechanism maps may be particularly useful for less experienced learners and/or those less familiar clinical or pathophysiologic concepts.

SUMMARY

The ICU represents a challenging clinical environment with numerous distractions and a large volume of clinical data to identify and process. Engaging in effective and efficient critical thinking skills is an important component of achieving accurate clinical reasoning and for making appropriate clinical decisions. Identifying, defining, and describing models of cognition, such as the dual process theory of cognition, can promote metacognition, a core component of critical thinking. Furthermore, naming, defining, describing, and understanding cognitive biases such as anchoring and availability bias is an important step in promoting critical thinking in the ICU. Educational strategies that use concept or mechanism mapping in the ICU can help to diagnose disorganized thinking and reinforce key connections and important clinical and pathophysiologic concepts. Critical thinking requires cognitive effort and focus, which can be difficult in the busy ICU setting, but is essential to reduce cognitive error. By using these educational strategies, faculty can help promote effective critical thinking on the ICU team.

CLINICS CARE POINTS

- Critical thinking is variably defined in the literature but is best described as applying higher cognitive skills such as conceptualization, analysis, and evaluation of medical information in a manner that results in precise, consistent, logical, and appropriate clinical decisions and actions.

- Awareness of the dual process model of clinical reasoning and relevant cognitive biases can increase metacognitive practices and potentially decrease the risk of falling victim to cognitive biases and committing diagnostic errors.
- Think-pair-share is an effective educational strategy to increase engagement and leverage critical thinking skills in the conference room or clinical setting.
- Concept or mechanism maps improve self-perceived reasoning and teamwork skills, as well as performance on summative examinations, and can be used in teaching concepts or topics to clinical learners.
- Prioritizing "how" or "why" questions in the clinical setting can emphasize analytical reasoning and encourage learners to go beyond superficial understanding of medical topics or concepts.

DISCLOSURE

The authors have nothing to disclose.

REFERENCES

1. Winters B, Custer J, Galvagno SM, et al. Diagnostic errors in the intensive care unit: a systematic review of autopsy studies. BMJ Qual Saf 2012;21(11):894–902.
2. Croskerry P. The importance of cognitive errors in diagnosis and strategies to minimize them. Acad Med J Assoc Am Med Coll 2003;78(8):775–80.
3. Donchin Y, Gopher D, Olin M, et al. A look into the nature and causes of human errors in the intensive care unit. Crit Care Med 1995;23(2):294–300.
4. Moyen E, Camiré E, Stelfox HT. Clinical review: Medication errors in critical care. Crit Care 2008;12(2):208.
5. Bergl PA, Nanchal RS, Singh H. Diagnostic error in the critically Ill: defining the problem and exploring next steps to advance intensive care unit safety. Ann Am Thorac Soc 2018;15(8):903–7.
6. Zwaan L, de Bruijne M, Wagner C, et al. Patient record review of the incidence, consequences, and causes of diagnostic adverse events. Arch Intern Med 2010;170(12):1015–21.
7. Wilcox ME, Harrison DA, Patel A, et al. Higher ICU capacity strain is associated with increased acute mortality in closed ICUs. Crit Care Med 2020;48(5):709–16.
8. Rewa OG, Stelfox HT, Ingolfsson A, et al. Indicators of intensive care unit capacity strain: a systematic review. Crit Care Lond Engl 2018;22(1):86.
9. Kane-Gill SL, O'Connor MF, Rothschild JM, et al. Technologic distractions (Part 1): summary of approaches to manage alert quantity with intent to reduce alert fatigue and suggestions for alert fatigue metrics. Crit Care Med 2017;45(9):1481–8.
10. Kahlke R, Eva K. Constructing critical thinking in health professional education. Perspect Med Educ 2018;7(3):156–65.
11. Defining critical thinking. Available at: https://www.criticalthinking.org/pages/defining-critical-thinking/766. Accessed April 26, 2021.
12. [C01] What is critical thinking?. Available at: https://philosophy.hku.hk/think/critical/ct.php. Accessed April 26, 2021.
13. Berg C, Philipp R, Taff SD. Scoping review of critical thinking literature in healthcare education. Occup Ther Health Care 2021;1–18.
14. Facione PA. Critical thinking: what it is and why it counts. San Jose, CA: Academic Press; 2011.

15. Huang GC, Newman LR, Schwartzstein RM. Critical thinking in health professions education: summary and consensus statements of the Millennium Conference 2011. Teach Learn Med 2014;26(1):95–102.
16. Krupat E, Sprague JM, Wolpaw D, et al. Thinking critically about critical thinking: ability, disposition or both? Med Educ 2011;45(6):625–35.
17. Papp KK, Huang GC, Lauzon Clabo LM, et al. Milestones of critical thinking: a developmental model for medicine and nursing. Acad Med J Assoc Am Med Coll 2014;89(5):715–20.
18. Croskerry P. Clinical cognition and diagnostic error: applications of a dual process model of reasoning. Adv Health Sci Educ Theory Pract 2009;14(Suppl 1): 27–35.
19. Imel S. Metacognitive skills for adult learning. Trends and issues alert. 2002. Available at: https://eric.ed.gov/?id=ED469264. Accessed April 25, 2021.
20. Graber ML, Franklin N, Gordon R. Diagnostic error in internal medicine. Arch Intern Med 2005;165(13):1493–9.
21. Prince MJ, Felder RM. Inductive teaching and learning methods: definitions, comparisons, and research bases. J Eng Educ 2006;95(2):123–38.
22. Bowen JL. Educational strategies to promote clinical diagnostic reasoning. N Engl J Med 2006;355(21):2217–25.
23. Saposnik G, Redelmeier D, Ruff CC, et al. Cognitive biases associated with medical decisions: a systematic review. BMC Med Inform Decis Mak 2016;16.
24. Brewer NT, Chapman GB, Schwartz JA, et al. The influence of irrelevant anchors on the judgments and choices of doctors and patients. Med Decis Mak Int J Soc Med Decis Mak 2007;27(2):203–11.
25. Kassirer JP. Teaching clinical reasoning: case-based and coached. Acad Med J Assoc Am Med Coll 2010;85(7):1118–24.
26. McDonald KM, Matesic B, Contopoulos-Ioannidis DG, et al. Patient safety strategies targeted at diagnostic errors: a systematic review. Ann Intern Med 2013; 158(5 Pt 2):381–9.
27. Graber ML, Mathew A. Performance of a web-based clinical diagnosis support system for internists. J Gen Intern Med 2008;23(Suppl 1):37–40.
28. Mamede S, van Gog T, van den Berge K, et al. Effect of availability bias and reflective reasoning on diagnostic accuracy among internal medicine residents. J Am Med Assoc 2010;304(11):1198–203.
29. Croskerry P. From mindless to mindful practice–cognitive bias and clinical decision making. N Engl J Med 2013;368(26):2445–8.
30. Dunlop M, Schwartzstein RM. Reducing diagnostic error in the intensive care unit. Engaging uncertainty when teaching clinical reasoning. SCH 2020;1(4): 364–71.
31. Connors GR, Siner JM. Clinical reasoning and risk in the intensive care unit. Clin Chest Med 2015;36(3):449–59.
32. Croskerry P. The feedback sanction. Acad Emerg Med Off J Soc Acad Emerg Med 2000;7(11):1232–8.
33. Torralba KD, Jose D, Byrne J. Psychological safety, the hidden curriculum, and ambiguity in medicine. Clin Rheumatol 2020;39(3):667–71.
34. Joynt GM, Wong W-T, Ling L, et al. Medical students and professionalism - do the hidden curriculum and current role models fail our future doctors? Med Teach 2018;40(4):395–9.
35. Remtulla R, Hagana A, Houbby N, et al. Exploring the barriers and facilitators of psychological safety in primary care teams: a qualitative study. BMC Health Serv Res 2021;21(1):269.

36. Mulder H, Ter Braak E, Chen HC, et al. Addressing the hidden curriculum in the clinical workplace: a practical tool for trainees and faculty. Med Teach 2019;41(1): 36–43.
37. Trowbridge RL. Twelve tips for teaching avoidance of diagnostic errors. Med Teach 2008;30(5):496–500.
38. Huang GC, Kriegel G, Wheaton C, et al. Implementation of diagnostic pauses in the ambulatory setting. BMJ Qual Saf 2018;27(6):492–7.
39. Kasick RT, Melvin JE, Perera ST, et al. A diagnostic time-out to improve differential diagnosis in pediatric abdominal pain. Diagn Berl Ger 2019. https://doi.org/10.1515/dx-2019-0054.
40. Hautz WE, Kämmer JE, Schauber SK, et al. Diagnostic performance by medical students working individually or in teams. J Am Med Assoc 2015;313(3):303–4.
41. Kämmer JE, Hautz WE, Herzog SM, et al. The potential of collective intelligence in emergency medicine: pooling medical students' independent decisions improves diagnostic performance. Med Decis Mak Int J Soc Med Decis Mak 2017;37(6):715–24.
42. Wolf M, Krause J, Carney PA, et al. Collective intelligence meets medical decision-making: the collective outperforms the best radiologist. PLoS One 2015;10(8):e0134269.
43. McTiGHE J, Lyman FT. Cueing thinking in the classroom: the promise of theory-embedded tools. Educ Leadersh 1988;8.
44. Krupat E, Richards JB, Sullivan AM, et al. Assessing the effectiveness of case-based collaborative learning via randomized controlled trial. Acad Med J Assoc Am Med Coll 2016;91(5):723–9.
45. Carpenter PB, Poliak A, Wang L, et al. Improved performance in and preference for using think-pair-share in a flipped classroom. Med Educ 2020;54(5):449–50.
46. Rao SP, DiCarlo SE. Peer instruction improves performance on quizzes. Adv Physiol Educ 2000;24(1):51–5.
47. Lom B. Classroom Activities: simple strategies to incorporate student-centered activities within undergraduate science lectures. J Undergrad Neurosci Educ 2012;11(1):A64–71.
48. Hausmann JS, Schwartzstein RM. Using questions to enhance rheumatology education. Arthritis Care Res 2019;71(10):1304–9.
49. Neher JO, Gordon KC, Meyer B, et al. A five-step "microskills" model of clinical teaching. J Am Board Fam Pract 1992;5(4):419–24.
50. Wolpaw T, Papp KK, Bordage G. Using SNAPPS to facilitate the expression of clinical reasoning and uncertainties: a randomized comparison group trial. Acad Med J Assoc Am Med Coll 2009;84(4):517–24.
51. Ogdie AR, Reilly JB, Pang WG, et al. Seen through their eyes: residents' reflections on the cognitive and contextual components of diagnostic errors in medicine. Acad Med J Assoc Am Med Coll 2012;87(10):1361–7.
52. Novak JD, Gowin DB. Learning how to learn. Cambridge University Press; 1984.
53. Fischer K, Sullivan AM, Krupat E, et al. Assessing the effectiveness of using mechanistic concept maps in case-based collaborative learning. Acad Med J Assoc Am Med Coll 2019;94(2):208–12.
54. West DC, Pomeroy JR, Park JK, et al. Critical thinking in graduate medical education: a role for concept mapping assessment? J Am Med Assoc 2000;284(9): 1105–10.
55. Irvine LM. Can concept mapping be used to promote meaningful learning in nurse education? J Adv Nurs 1995;21(6):1175–9.

56. Hung C-H, Lin C-Y. Using concept mapping to evaluate knowledge structure in problem-based learning. BMC Med Educ 2015;15:212.
57. Veronese C, Richards JB, Pernar L, et al. A randomized pilot study of the use of concept maps to enhance problem-based learning among first-year medical students. Med Teach 2013;35(9):e1478–84.
58. Baliga SS, Walvekar PR, Mahantshetti GJ. Concept map as a teaching and learning tool for medical students. J Educ Health Promot 2021;10:35.
59. Silva Ezequiel O da, Cerrato Tibirica SH, Damasio Moutinho IL, et al. Medical students' critical thinking assessment with collaborative concept maps in a blended educational Strategy. Educ Health Abingdon Engl 2019;32(3):127–30.
60. Slieman TA, Camarata T. Case-based group learning using concept maps to achieve multiple educational objectives and behavioral outcomes. J Med Educ Curric Dev 2019;6. 2382120519872510.

Enhancing Diagnosis Through Technology
Decision Support, Artificial Intelligence, and Beyond

Robert El-Kareh, MD, MPH, MS[a],*, Dean F. Sittig, PhD[b]

KEYWORDS

- Clinical decision support • Diagnostic decision support • Data visualization
- Clinical informatics

KEY POINTS

- Critical care settings are well-suited to diagnostic clinical decision support because of high clinical acuity, time pressure, and large volumes and variety of data.
- There are multiple types of clinical decision support that are helpful at many points in the diagnostic process in critical care settings.
- Evolving approaches using artificial intelligence, machine learning, and natural language processing hold promise to improve patient care and provider experiences.
- Diagnostic decision support interventions require careful integration into clinical workflows to have the highest impact and avoid unintended consequences.

INTRODUCTION

Critical care settings are complex environments that are well-suited for diagnostic clinical decision support (CDS). First, the patients are critically ill and decisions need to be made quickly to avoid rapid patient deterioration, morbidity, and mortality.[1] Second, the clinical issues are often complex with involvement of multiple organ systems and surgical procedures.[2] Finally, the variety, velocity, and volume of the data generated in these settings is large, pushing the limits of human cognitive abilities to process all the relevant data in a timely fashion. For these reasons, CDS is a set of promising approaches that can allow technology to partner with clinicians to provide high-quality, safe, and effective care.

[a] University of California, San Diego, 9500 Gilman Drive, #0881 La Jolla, CA 92093-0881, USA;
[b] School of Biomedical Informatics, The University of Texas Health Science Center at Houston, UT-Memorial Hermann Center for Healthcare Quality & Safety, Houston, TX 77030, USA
* Corresponding author.
E-mail address: relkareh@health.ucsd.edu
Twitter: @DeanSittig (D.F.S.)

Crit Care Clin 38 (2022) 129–139
https://doi.org/10.1016/j.ccc.2021.08.004
0749-0704/22/© 2021 Elsevier Inc. All rights reserved.

TYPES OF CLINICAL DECISION SUPPORT

A CDS system is defined as one that "provides clinicians, staff, patients, or other individuals with knowledge and person-specific information, intelligently filtered or presented at appropriate times, to enhance health and health care."[3] The breadth of this definition encompasses a wide range of potential systems. Wright and colleagues[4] developed a taxonomy of CDS interventions that spans this range. In **Table 1**, we briefly introduce those categories with direct relevance to diagnostic decision support.

CATEGORIES OF DIAGNOSTIC DECISIONS APPLICATIONS OF CLINICAL DECISION SUPPORT
Diagnostic Tasks in Critical Care

The diagnostic process in critical care involves multiple different activities as described elsewhere in this issue. **Fig. 1** shows one potential model to organize these activities into five broader categories. Each of these diagnostic steps has the potential to be supported by different types of CDS and we describe a few examples to highlight these possibilities, recognizing that evolving CDS capabilities set the stage for ongoing innovation.

Recognize indication for intensive care unit
The first step to appropriate care in intensive care units (ICUs) is to recognize the indication for ICU admission. When patients require ICU care at their initial presentation, this triage requires an accurate assessment of illness severity during the initial evaluation.

Table 1	
Types of clinical decision support for diagnosis	
Type of CDS	**Description**
Order facilitators	These systems provide grouped sets of orders to streamline commonly ordered items. In addition, systems may request additional information from providers to ensure the proper order is initially selected.
Point-of-care alerts and reminders	These systems may alert providers to specific information using interruptive of passive means, depending on urgency. Examples of potential uses include prompting consideration of specific diagnostic tests, raising awareness of potential complications or interactions, and highlighting critical test results.
Relevant information display	These displays may be targeted, such as displaying renal function when ordering a contrast-enhanced imaging study. They may also include more sophisticated data aggregation and visualizations that bring together several data elements to allow clinicians to see patterns and understand the patient's current status and trajectory.
Expert systems	These systems provide complex decision support using a wide range of electronic data. Examples include differential diagnosis generators and risk and prognosis models.
Workflow support	These interventions include support, such as templates to facilitate reliable processes. Examples include support for registry functions across multiple patients and documentation aids.

Data from Wright A, Sittig DF, Ash JS, et al. Development and evaluation of a comprehensive clinical decision support taxonomy: comparison of front-end tools in commercial and internally developed electronic health record systems. J Am Med Inform Assoc. 2011;18(3):232-242.

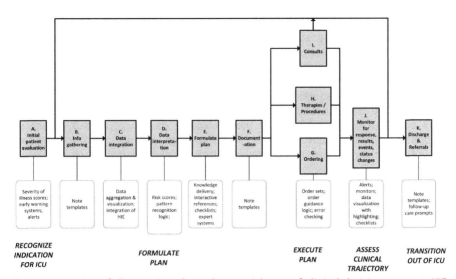

Fig. 1. Categories of diagnostic tasks and potential uses of clinical decision support. HIE, health information exchange; ICU, intensive care unit.

This triage is supported by illness-specific and/or general severity of illness scores. Illness-specific scores (eg, CURB65 for community-acquired pneumonia[5]) can perform well in targeted scenarios, but performance is somewhat variable.[6,7] General severity of illness scores and early warning systems (eg, APACHE IV,[8] pSOFA,[9] SIRS,[10] MEWS[11]) characterize overall physiologic derangements and have also shown mixed results when implemented into workflows.[6,12] However, if validated through well-designed studies, data-driven triaging tools may help ensure that critically ill patients are brought to the attention of ICU teams soon after initial presentation.

Another high-risk group of critically ill patients is those who do not require ICU level of care at initial presentation to the hospital, but deteriorate during their stay. Early recognition of this deterioration is crucial to prompt intervention to rescue these patients. Rapid response teams have been instituted to extend critical care expertise outside of the ICU. Failure to activate the rapid response team is one of the biggest contributors to failure to rescue.[13] As with severity of illness scores for initial presentation to the hospital, several data-driven deterioration scores have been developed for hospitalized patients. These systems for early detection of deterioration within the hospital have promise, but the true impact on outcomes remains unclear.[14,15]

For the initial severity of illness models and the deterioration scores, the scores are most useful when integrated directly into electronic health records (EHRs).[16] The score may be presented in the overview of groups of patients for prioritizing evaluation. In addition, the scores could be used to trigger specific alerts to prompt consideration of additional diagnostic and therapeutic interventions. For example, a general deterioration score can be shown as a column on a patient list and sorted to help teams see higher-scoring patients earlier in the day. These scores may also trigger "proactive rounding" by rapid response teams with the goal of preempting the need to transfer patients to a higher level of care.

Formulate plan

Once the patient has been triaged for evaluation for ICU admission, that evaluation requires a rapid collection of relevant clinical data. Providers face significant challenges gathering these data because they are often scattered across many sources and not well-organized.[17] When surveyed about chart review workflow during initial evaluation, half of providers described their process as haphazard or disorganized. In addition, they noted that their diagnostic and therapeutic strategy was often established by chart review alone.[18] Findings such as these highlight opportunities to improve data aggregation, summarization, and visualization for critical care providers. Efforts are underway to develop data displays that are better aligned to clinician cognitive processes,[19,20] but these displays have not yet had widespread adoption. Documentation templates have also been used to improved data gathering by prompting clinicians to obtain a complete set of clinical data for initial evaluation. In addition, these templates can automatically import data from the EHR into the note to facilitate review.

Beyond merely obtaining all relevant clinical data, critical care providers must integrate and interpret these data to properly assess the patient's current clinical state and trajectory and to drive appropriate diagnostic and therapeutic interventions. Well-designed data displays can highlight important information[21] and enable interactive exploration of clinical data.[22–24] The latter capability is important because there is sufficient variability among critically ill patients to require a personalized approach to data review.[23] Studies in simulated environments have shown significant impact, but translation of these results into real-world settings has remained elusive.[22] At least one study using a simulated EHR environment demonstrated decreased search time and fewer errors using a problem-oriented view of clinical data.[25]

A key step in diagnostic evaluations is to have an appropriately broad differential diagnosis (prioritized list of potential diagnoses) early in the process. Different forms of CDS are used to facilitate the creation of the differential diagnosis. The organization may provide links within the clinician workflow to curated clinical references (eg, DynaMed, UpToDate) to enable point-of-care review of relevant knowledge and diagnostic guidelines. Checklists are another potential intervention and several critical care–specific checklists have been created.[26] These checklists can be linked as references or some may be incorporated directly into the assessment and plan sections of documentation templates.

Expert systems can also be used to provide additional support for development of differential diagnoses and for identifying the additional clinical information that would help narrow down the diagnosis (ie, the best next test). Briefly, expert systems rely on a large corpus of "if-then-else" rules derived from clinical experts and the scientific literature to help clinicians identify the correct diagnosis.

Preliminary data suggest an expert system is useful in the general medical inpatient setting,[27] but robust evaluation within critical care settings is currently unavailable. Better integration of expert systems into EHRs could help reduce the data entry requirement that is often cited as a barrier to their use.

When infections are considered, one aspect of diagnosis is to consider the potential causative organisms. Expert systems are used to ensure that the appropriate spectrum of potential infectious causes is considered and consequently that appropriate antimicrobial therapy is selected. One such system was shown to improve patient outcomes and lower costs.[28]

Critical care settings, as with many others, often involve a substantial number of care handoffs. Therefore, proper documentation of clinical reasoning and certainty around the working diagnosis is an important step to continuity of care across these transitions. Documentation templates have been used to prompt the recording of diagnostic reasoning, although there is limited published literature describing their impact in critical care settings.

Execute plan

CDS has a clear role in supporting the execution of diagnostic plans. One function of CDS during this stage is to ensure that the intended work-up includes all relevant orders. Order facilitators, such as indication-based order sets, can serve as evidence-based or standard of care collections of related orders to avoid inadvertent oversight. For example, these order sets can include related diagnostic tests for samples collected during procedures, such as paracentesis, thoracentesis, or lumbar puncture, or a set of tests to work up anemia. These order sets may also include consultations to specialists in certain circumstances.[29]

In addition to prompting consideration of tests, CDS may also be used to highlight potentially low-yield or inappropriate tests as part of diagnostic stewardship programs. Examples include alerts highlighting when laboratory tests are ordered more frequently than likely to be clinically useful[30,31] and when tests for *Clostridioides difficile* are ordered on patients lacking clear indications.[32] Initial studies of these approaches have suggested decreased test use is achieved without adversely affecting patient outcomes.

CDS during ordering can also be used to suggest alternative tests that may be more appropriate for that particular patient. This approach has been used for advanced imaging studies. Based on the indication for the test and patient-specific criteria, the system can present the ordering provider with alternative imaging that may be more appropriate.[33] It has yet to be seen whether this approach leads to substantial changes in imaging or whether clinicians alter their interaction with the system to satisfy the appropriateness check and to obtain their initially desired test.

Recognize events and changes in clinical status

The large volume of data collected on patients while they are in the ICU presents a challenge to the care teams. They must process these data to promptly respond to new test results, clinical events, and changes in patients' status. A key role for CDS is to facilitate this process. The previously mentioned approaches to improve data summarization and visualization are likely to be helpful in enabling clinicians to recognize important events and changes in status.[19–21]

Diagnosis in intensive care settings involves many team members and therefore the CDS systems can target a wide range of providers. Nurses likely have the most time directly at patients' bedsides and are key partners in diagnostic processes. The effectiveness of CDS for ICU nurses has not been fully evaluated. This area represents a substantial opportunity to support diagnostic excellence.[34] One approach that has been well-studied is the use of daily screening checklists (often facilitated within EHRs) for the identification of delirium in the ICU,[35] although early diagnosis of this condition does not always lead to effective intervention.[36]

Respiratory therapists are also crucial members of the diagnostic team in ICUs. There is substantial overlap between diagnosis and optimal treatment of patients receiving invasive and noninvasive ventilation. For example, adjustment of ventilator settings involves diagnosis of an opportunity to wean ventilation or a need for adjustment to provide effective therapy. Systems have been developed to analyze mechanical ventilation pressures, flows, and settings, and make recommendations to providers regarding potential patient-specific adjustments.[37,38]

Checklists can represent a manual process to identify patients at high risk of events. Developing models that automatically calculate risk scores based on EHR data can add powerful options for early detection of important conditions in ICUs. These models may be based on traditional methods, such as logistic regression. Examples include models to identify risk of acute respiratory distress syndrome after trauma[39] or development of acute kidney injury.[40]

More complex artificial intelligence predictive algorithms have the potential to improve the performance of these predictions. As Yu and colleagues[41] describe, "with deep-learning algorithms, raw patient-monitoring data could be better used to avoid information overload and alert overload while enabling more accurate clinical prediction and timely decision-making." These approaches are being applied to predict a variety of intensive care conditions, such as hypotension[2] or the onset of sepsis.[42] The scores from checklists or predictive models can be shown directly to providers and used to trigger alerts or additional protocols.

Transition out of intensive care unit

Similar to other settings in the hospital, the transition at the time of discharge from the ICU requires effective communication of the status of the diagnostic work-up and any diagnosis-related follow-up required.[43] This communication should involve the patient and subsequent providers.[43] The transfer of ICU patients to the general wards is a vulnerable process and is often not standardized.[44] From a CDS standpoint, documentation templates have been used to improve the completeness of information transfer.[44] Although opportunities remain to improve information transfer during this transition, there is a lack of evidence regarding the most effective support of this process.[45]

Diagnostic feedback for calibration

We expect clinicians to improve the calibration of their diagnostic decision-making with experience. This process requires ongoing feedback of the outcomes of their decisions, but this feedback is often lacking.[46–48] Improving patient data visualization to enable clinicians to "close the loop" on their decisions has the potential to meet this need and improve diagnostic performance over time. One example of such a system includes provider-specific dashboards that highlight recent patients and their outcomes after care was handed off to other providers, such as the Post-Handoff Reports of Outcomes (PHAROS) system.[49] In an ICU setting, such a system could be modified to highlight specific downstream outcomes or events of interest, including return to ICU, urgent/emergent surgical procedures, death, and so forth. These dashboards could be coupled with dedicated time to reflect on the care of recent patients to identify individual and organizational opportunities for improvement.

IMPLEMENTATION ISSUES

CDS is one component of a complex care environment.[50] In addition to the quality of the data and the accuracy of any predictions, the implementation of CDS systems can greatly affect their impact.[51] Prior experience with CDS across a variety of settings has provided best practices regarding the development of CDS, encapsulated by the "Five Rights of CDS" (**Table 2**).[52]

As artificial intelligence, machine learning, and other predictive models become more widespread, one key aspect of increasing their impact is to ensure that the output of these models is directly tied to a specific clinical workflow.[53] That is, if a patient is found to be at risk of a significant clinical outcome, who gets notified and what action is then taken? Without clear delineation of these aspects of the workflow, the identification of high-risk scenarios may not lead to improved patient care.

Given the complexities of incorporating CDS systems into ICU settings and their potential impact on providers and patients, having clear governance of CDS portfolios is recommended.[54] This governance involves careful consideration of how new CDS will

Table 2	
The five rights of clinical decision support	
Component	Description
Right information	Evidence-based guidance, response to clinical need
Right person	Targeting decision-makers, including the patient
Right CDS format	For example, order sets, flow-sheets, dashboards, patient lists
Right channel	For example, EHR, mobile device, patient portal
Right time in workflow	For decision making or action

Data from Osheroff JA, Teich JM, Levick D, et al. Improving outcomes with clinical decision support: an implementer's guide. CRC Press; 2012.

affect the care environment and its participants before implementation. It is also important to develop tools and processes to monitor CDS interventions over time and to promptly adjust, optimize, or deactivate them if the clinical scenarios warrant.[54]

FUTURE DIRECTIONS AND OPPORTUNITIES FOR CLINICAL DECISION SUPPORT IN INTENSIVE CARE UNITS

Intensive care settings are well-suited for ongoing innovation and additional diagnostic CDS interventions. Artificial intelligence and various forms of predictive modeling using the full spectrum of available electronic data are likely to play a prominent role in this area. Some use cases may involve systems to suggest specific diagnoses based on full record review[55] and models to better identify and highlight unexpected clinical trajectories. Much of the information related to clinician assessments and reasoning is contained in free text notes. For this reason, more extensive use of natural language processing is important to push diagnostic CDS forward.[41,56]

There are continued opportunities to improve the display of patient-specific relevant information to reduce the cognitive load on providers and facilitate faster and more accurate clinical assessments. In particular, it will be important to effectively display and model the temporal aspect of diagnostic information. Potential functionality to support this goal includes display of trends with highlighting of substantial changes in vital signs, laboratory values, or other numerical trends[23] and using established interactive features, such as graphical zoom, pan, and filtering.[24] One specific area that may benefit from this type of approach is the assessment of intravascular fluid status and subsequent fluid management.[57,58]

To support reflective practice and ongoing diagnostic calibration, CDS systems should be developed to provide systematic feedback of diagnostic outcomes to clinicians. Functionality that has been used to support clinical care and reporting can be harnessed to augment ongoing learning. Improvement opportunities from the systems can be provided at the individual clinician and organizational levels.

SUMMARY

Patient care in intensive care environments is complex, time-sensitive, and data-rich, factors that make these settings particularly well-suited to CDS. A wide range of CDS interventions have been used in ICU environments. However, robust data on their impact on patient outcomes are often lacking. The field is in need of well-designed studies to identify the most effective CDS approaches. The continued evolution of artificial intelligence and machine learning models may reduce the information-overload and enable teams to take better advantage of the large volume of patient data available to them. It is vital to effectively integrate new CDS into clinical workflows and to align closely with the cognitive processes of frontline clinicians.

ACKNOWLEDGMENTS

Dr. El-Kareh's work was funded by the National Library of Medicine (K22LM011435) and the Gordon and Betty Moore Foundation.

DISCLOSURE

The authors have nothing to disclose.

REFERENCES

1. Belard A, Buchman T, Forsberg J, et al. Precision diagnosis: a view of the clinical decision support systems (CDSS) landscape through the lens of critical care. J Clin Monit Comput 2017;31(2):261–71.
2. Pirracchio R, Cohen MJ, Malenica I, et al. Big data and targeted machine learning in action to assist medical decision in the ICU. Anaesth Crit Care Pain Med 2019; 38(4):377–84.
3. HealthIT.gov. Available at: https://www.healthit.gov/topic/safety/clinical-decision-support. Accessed April 10, 2021.
4. Wright A, Sittig DF, Ash JS, et al. Development and evaluation of a comprehensive clinical decision support taxonomy: comparison of front-end tools in commercial and internally developed electronic health record systems. J Am Med Inform Assoc 2011;18(3):232–42.
5. Lim WS, van der Eerden MM, Laing R, et al. Defining community acquired pneumonia severity on presentation to hospital: an international derivation and validation study. Thorax 2003;58(5):377–82.
6. Downey CL, Tahir W, Randell R, et al. Strengths and limitations of early warning scores: a systematic review and narrative synthesis. Int J Nurs Stud 2017;76: 106–19.
7. Makam AN, Nguyen OK, Auerbach AD. Diagnostic accuracy and effectiveness of automated electronic sepsis alert systems: a systematic review. J Hosp Med 2015;10(6):396–402.
8. Zimmerman JE, Kramer AA, McNair DS, et al. Acute physiology and chronic health evaluation (Apache) IV: hospital mortality assessment for today's critically ill patients. Crit Care Med 2006;34(5):1297–310.
9. Shime N, Kawasaki T, Nakagawa S. Proposal of a new pediatric sequential organ failure assessment score for possible validation. Pediatr Crit Care Med 2017; 18(1):98–9.
10. Bone RC, Balk RA, Cerra FB, et al. Definitions for sepsis and organ failure and guidelines for the use of innovative therapies in sepsis. Chest 1992;101(6): 1644–55.
11. Subbe CP, Kruger M, Rutherford P, et al. Validation of a modified early warning score in medical admissions. QJM 2001;94(10):521–6.
12. Wulff A, Montag S, Marschollek M, et al. Clinical decision-support systems for detection of systemic inflammatory response syndrome, sepsis, and septic shock in critically ill patients: a systematic review. Methods Inf Med 2019;58:e43–57.
13. Bassily-Marcus A. Early detection of deteriorating patients: leveraging clinical informatics to improve outcome*. Crit Care Med 2014;42(4):976–8.

14. Smith MEB, Chiovaro JC, O'Neil M, et al. Early warning system scores for clinical deterioration in hospitalized patients: a systematic review. Ann Am Thorac Soc 2014;11(9):1454–65.

15. Evans RS, Kuttler KG, Simpson KJ, et al. Automated detection of physiologic deterioration in hospitalized patients. J Am Med Inform Assoc 2015;22(2):350–60.

16. Aakre C, Franco PM, Ferreyra M, et al. Prospective validation of a near real-time EHR-integrated automated SOFA score calculator. Int J Med Inform 2017;103:1–6.

17. Pickering BW, Gajic O, Ahmed A, et al. Data utilization for medical decision making at the time of patient Admission to ICU. Crit Care Med 2013;41(6):1502–10.

18. Nolan ME, Cartin-Ceba R, Moreno-Franco P, et al. A multisite survey study of EMR review habits, information needs, and display preferences among medical ICU clinicians evaluating new patients. Appl Clin Inform 2017;8(4):1197–207.

19. Lasko TA, Owens DA, Fabbri D, et al. User-centered clinical display design issues for inpatient providers. Appl Clin Inform 2020;11(05):700–9.

20. Glicksberg BS, Oskotsky B, Thangaraj PM, et al. PatientExploreR: an extensible application for dynamic visualization of patient clinical history from electronic health records in the OMOP common data model. Bioinformatics 2019;35(21):4515–8.

21. King AJ, Cooper GF, Clermont G, et al. Using machine learning to selectively highlight patient information. J Biomed Inform 2019;100:10.

22. Waller RG, Wright MC, Segall N, et al. Novel displays of patient information in critical care settings: a systematic review. J Am Med Inform Assoc 2019;26(5):479–89.

23. Calzoni L, Clermont G, Cooper GF, et al. Graphical presentations of clinical data in a learning electronic medical record. Appl Clin Inform 2020;11(04):680–91.

24. West VL, Borland D, Hammond WE. Innovative information visualization of electronic health record data: a systematic review. J Am Med Inform Assoc 2015;22(2):330–9.

25. Semanik MG, Kleinschmidt PC, Wright A, et al. Impact of a problem-oriented view on clinical data retrieval. J Am Med Inform Assoc 2021;28(5):899–906.

26. Barwise A, Garcia-Arguello L, Dong Y, et al. Checklist for Early Recognition and Treatment of Acute Illness (CERTAIN): evolution of a content management system for point-of-care clinical decision support. BMC Med Inform Decis Mak 2016;16:10.

27. Elkin PL, Liebow M, Bauer BA, et al. The introduction of a diagnostic decision support system (DXplain) into the workflow of a teaching hospital service can decrease the cost of service for diagnostically challenging Diagnostic Related Groups (DRGs). Int J Med Inform 2010;79(11):772–7.

28. Evans RS, Pestotnik SL, Classen DC, et al. A computer-assisted management program for antibiotics and other antiinfective agents. N Engl J Med 1998;338(4):232–8.

29. Wright A, Sittig DF, Carpenter JD, et al. Order sets in computerized physician order entry systems: an analysis of seven sites. AMIA Annu Symp Proc 2010;2010:892–6.

30. Levick DL, Stern G, Meyerhoefer CD, et al. Reducing unnecessary testing in a CPOE system through implementation of a targeted CDS intervention. BMC Med Inform Decis Mak 2013;13:7.

31. Pageler NM, Franzon D, Longhurst CA, et al. Embedding time-limited laboratory orders within computerized provider order entry reduces laboratory utilization. Pediatr Crit Care Med 2013;14(4):413–9.
32. Dunn AN, Radakovich N, Ancker JS, et al. The impact of clinical decision support alerts on *Clostridioides difficile* testing: a systematic review. Clin Infect Dis 2021;72(6):987–94.
33. Hussey PS, Timbie JW, Burgette LF, et al. Appropriateness of advanced diagnostic imaging ordering before and after implementation of clinical decision support systems. JAMA 2015;313(21):2181–2.
34. Nibbelink CW, Young JR, Carrington JM, et al. Informatics solutions for application of decision-making skills. Crit Care Nurs Clin North Am 2018;30(2):237–46.
35. Gusmao-Flores D, Salluh JIF, Chalhub RA, et al. The confusion assessment method for the intensive care unit (CAM-ICU) and intensive care delirium screening checklist (ICDSC) for the diagnosis of delirium: a systematic review and meta-analysis of clinical studies. Crit Care 2012;16(4):10.
36. Riker RR, Fraser GL. Delirium-beyond the CAM-ICU. Crit Care Med 2020;48(1):134–6.
37. Khemani RG, Hotz JC, Sward KA, et al. The role of computer-based clinical decision support systems to deliver protective mechanical ventilation. Curr Opin Crit Care 2020;26(1):73–81.
38. Tams C, Stephan P, Euliano N, et al. Clinical decision support recommending ventilator settings during noninvasive ventilation. J Clin Monit Comput 2020;34(5):1043–9.
39. Watkins TR, Nathens AB, Cooke CR, et al. Acute respiratory distress syndrome after trauma: development and validation of a predictive model. Crit Care Med 2012;40(8):2295–303.
40. Sanchez-Pinto LN, Khemani RG. Development of a prediction model of early acute kidney injury in critically ill children using electronic health record data. Pediatr Crit Care Med 2016;17(6):508–15.
41. Yu KH, Beam AL, Kohane IS. Artificial intelligence in healthcare. Nat Biomed Eng 2018;2(10):719–31.
42. Desautels T, Calvert J, Hoffman J, et al. Prediction of sepsis in the intensive care unit with minimal electronic health record data: a machine learning approach. JMIR Med Inform 2016;4(3):e28.
43. Snow V, Beck D, Budnitz T, et al. Transitions of care consensus policy statement: American College of Physicians, Society of General Internal Medicine, Society of Hospital Medicine, American Geriatrics Society, American College of Emergency Physicians, and Society for Academic Emergency Medicine. J Hosp Med 2009;4(6):364–70.
44. Santhosh L, Lyons PG, Rojas JC, et al. Characterising ICU-ward handoffs at three academic medical centres: process and perceptions. BMJ Qual Saf 2019;28(8):627–34.
45. Co I, Hyzy RC. Lost in transition: a call to arms for better transition from ICU to hospital ward. Crit Care Med 2020;48(7):1075–6.
46. Bhat PN, Costello JM, Aiyagari R, et al. Diagnostic errors in paediatric cardiac intensive care. Cardiol Young 2018;28(5):675–82.
47. Shenvi EC, Feupe SF, Yang H, et al. Closing the loop": a mixed-methods study about resident learning from outcome feedback after patient handoffs. Diagnosis (Berl) 2018;5(4):235–42.

48. Cifra CL, Sittig DF, Singh H. Bridging the feedback gap: a sociotechnical approach to informing clinicians of patients' subsequent clinical course and outcomes. BMJ Qual Saf 2021;30(7):591–7.
49. Rudolf F, Pott E, Oyama L, El-Kareh R. Post handoff report of outcomes to facilitate patient follow-up and reflection for emergency medicine residents. The Diagnostic Error in Medicine 13th Annual International Conference. Virtual. Oct 19-21, 2020.
50. Sittig DF, Singh H. A new sociotechnical model for studying health information technology in complex adaptive healthcare systems. Qual Saf Health Care 2010;19(Suppl 3):i68–74.
51. Scheepers-Hoeks AMJ, Grouls RJ, Neef C, et al. Physicians' responses to clinical decision support on an intensive care unit: comparison of four different alerting methods. Artif Intell Med 2013;59(1):33–8.
52. Osheroff JA, Teich JM, Levick D, et al. Improving outcomes with clinical decision support: an implementer's guide. Boca Raton (FL): CRC Press; 2012.
53. Jung K, Kashyap S, Avati A, et al. A framework for making predictive models useful in practice. J Am Med Inform Assoc 2020;28(6):1149–58.
54. Wright A, Sittig DF, Ash JS, et al. Governance for clinical decision support: case studies and recommended practices from leading institutions. J Am Med Inform Assoc 2011;18(2):187–94.
55. Liang HY, Tsui BY, Ni H, et al. Evaluation and accurate diagnoses of pediatric diseases using artificial intelligence. Nat Med 2019;25(3):433–438.
56. Letourneau-Guillon L, Camirand D, Guilbert F, et al. Artificial intelligence applications for workflow, process optimization and predictive analytics. Neuroimaging Clin N Am 2020;30(4):E1–E15.
57. Bergmosera K, Pflanzl-Knizaceka L, Hafnera M, et al. Improving fluid management in critical care: towards the ICU of the future. In: Schreier G, Hayn D, editors. Health informatics meets ehealth: biomedical meets ehealth - from sensors to decisions, vol. 248. Amsterdam: Ios Press; 2018. p. 47–54.
58. Liu SQ, See KC, Ngiam KY, et al. Reinforcement learning for clinical decision support in critical care: comprehensive review. J Med Internet Res 2020;22(7):16.

A Research Agenda for Diagnostic Excellence in Critical Care Medicine

Christina L. Cifra, MD, MS[a],*, Jason W. Custer, MD[b,c],
James C. Fackler, MD[d,e]

KEYWORDS

- Critical care • Intensive care unit • Diagnosis • Diagnostic error • Misdiagnosis
- Patient safety

KEY POINTS

- Research to improve diagnosis in critical care medicine has accelerated with the increasing awareness of the burden and harms of diagnostic error among critically ill patients.
- Much work remains to fully elucidate the diagnostic process in critical care, which is fundamental to understanding how diagnostic errors occur in the intensive care unit.
- To achieve diagnostic excellence, interdisciplinary research is needed, adopting a balanced strategy of continued biomedical discovery while addressing the complex care delivery systems underpinning the diagnosis of critical illness.

INTRODUCTION

Diagnosing critically ill patients in the intensive care unit (ICU) is difficult. To arrive at an accurate and timely diagnosis, the intensivist must make sense of continuous data streams in the context of prior diagnostic labels to determine or confirm the underlying etiology of the patient's critical illness, while simultaneously searching for evidence of

Disclosure Statement and Funding Sources: All authors have no commercial or financial conflicts of interest to disclose. Dr Cifra is supported by the Agency for Healthcare Research and Quality (AHRQ) through a K08 grant (HS026965) and an internal start-up grant from the University of Iowa Carver College of Medicine Department of Pediatrics.
[a] Division of Critical Care, Department of Pediatrics, University of Iowa Carver College of Medicine, Iowa City, IA, USA; [b] Division of Critical Care, Department of Pediatrics, University of Maryland, 22 S Greene St, Baltimore, MD 21201, USA; [c] Medical Director of Patient Safety, University of Maryland Medical Center, Baltimore, MD, USA; [d] Division of Pediatric Anesthesia and Critical Care, Department of Anesthesiology and Critical Care Medicine, Johns Hopkins School of Medicine, Baltimore, MD, USA; [e] Johns Hopkins Charlotte R. Bloomberg Children's Center, 1800 Orleans St, Baltimore, MD 21287, USA
* Corresponding author. University of Iowa Hospitals and Clinics, 200 Hawkins Drive, 8600-M JCP, Iowa City, IA 52242.
E-mail address: christina-cifra@uiowa.edu
Twitter: @TinaCifra (C.L.C.); @jimfackler (J.C.F.)

impending physiologic disaster.[1] Critically ill patients often require life support, including mechanical ventilation and sedation, which make data gathering and interpretation more challenging.[2] The intensivist must incorporate evolving scientific progress in the definitions and diagnosis of commonly encountered syndromes and reconcile divergent opinions among ICU team members and consultants.[3] Clinicians must perform all of these tasks within the pressured ICU environment, which is known to increase the risk of clinician fatigue, emotional stress, and burnout.[4] As a result, diagnostic errors in the ICU are common and cause serious harm.[5,6,7,8,9]

The authors of the National Academies of Sciences, Engineering, and Medicine (NASEM) landmark report, *Improving Diagnosis in Health Care,* concluded that there is an urgent need for research on the diagnostic process and diagnostic error in medicine and listed high-yield areas for investigation.[10] Diagnostic safety experts have echoed this need for rigorous research.[11,12] Given this call and growing institutional and government support for diagnostic error research,[13,14] the time is ripe for investigators to broaden our understanding of diagnosis in critically ill patients. We present a research agenda geared toward diagnostic excellence in critical care medicine, advocating for a balanced strategy of continued biomedical discovery to improve the diagnosis of individual diseases while also addressing the complex care delivery systems underpinning the diagnostic process in critical care.

GAPS IN DIAGNOSIS RESEARCH IN CRITICAL CARE

The preceding decade brought about increasing knowledge of diagnostic errors in critical care. However, research on the diagnostic process and the development of effective interventions to improve diagnosis among critically ill patients remain underdeveloped. Autopsy studies remain a dominant source of data on ICU misdiagnoses despite autopsy rates of less than 50%.[5,6,15] There is little information available on the impact of diagnostic errors on critically ill patients, their families, and the ICU team, even though we know that misdiagnoses can contribute to death and disability,[5,6,16] have high financial costs resulting in billions of dollars in payouts for malpractice claims,[17,18] can be psychologically devastating to families,[19] and can negatively impact physicians' clinical practice, careers, and well-being.[20,21]

Because current avenues of research funding largely adopt a disease-focused approach, most research on diagnosis in the ICU is disease oriented. However, many diagnostic errors are likely underpinned by common diagnostic process missteps that require disease-agnostic approaches to address. It is impossible to understand fully how and why diagnostic errors occur in critically ill patients without studying the diagnostic process as a whole.[11] The fundamental components of diagnosis are rooted in, and affected by, the sociotechnical work environment of the ICU (**Fig. 1**).[1,22] We need to optimize the cognitive work of diagnosis as it occurs within the ICU work system and construct a conceptual model of critical care diagnosis to maximize the impact of disease-oriented diagnostic research and develop effective interventions toward diagnostic excellence.

A PROPOSED RESEARCH AGENDA
Defining the Diagnostic Process and the Burden of Diagnostic Error
The critical care diagnostic process
Improving diagnosis and preventing diagnostic error is only possible with a deep understanding of the diagnostic process, including its strengths and vulnerabilities. The diagnostic process is defined by NASEM as a complex, patient-centered, collaborative activity that involves information gathering and clinical reasoning with the goal

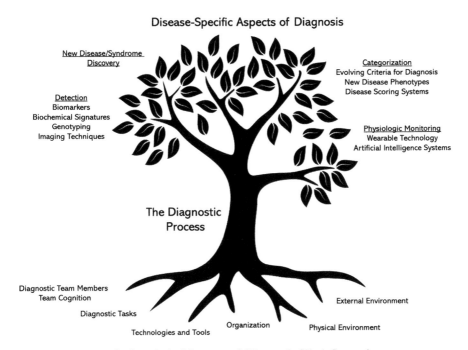

Disease-Specific Aspects of Diagnosis

New Disease/Syndrome Discovery

Detection
Biomarkers
Biochemical Signatures
Genotyping
Imaging Techniques

Categorization
Evolving Criteria for Diagnosis
New Disease Phenotypes
Disease Scoring Systems

Physiologic Monitoring
Wearable Technology
Artificial Intelligence Systems

The Diagnostic Process

Diagnostic Team Members
Team Cognition

Diagnostic Tasks

Technologies and Tools

Organization

External Environment

Physical Environment

Sociotechnical Aspects of Diagnosis (Work System)

Fig. 1. Disease-specific and sociotechnical aspects of the diagnostic process. Sociotechnical factors (work system) underpin the diagnostic process and must be considered alongside disease-specific considerations to improve the diagnosis of critical illness. (Illustration by Ani Rofiqah, https://thenounproject.com/.)

of explaining the patient's health problem. NASEM's model of the diagnostic process describes a patient seeking care for a health problem, clinicians undertaking an iterative process of information gathering and information integration/interpretation before arriving at a working diagnosis, treatment, response to treatment (serving as further information to confirm or revise the working diagnosis), and patient outcomes. The diagnostic process occurs over time and within the context of a larger health care work system, which in turn influences the process in many ways.[22] However, this model does not capture the complexity and challenges involved in critical care diagnosis fully, given the time and resource constraints as well as the severity of illness encountered unique to the critical care setting (**Fig. 2**).

Further research is needed to create a conceptual model of the diagnostic process specific to critical care. Each specific aspect should be studied to better elucidate the barriers and facilitators of timely and accurate diagnosis (**Table 1**). Some examples of important areas for future investigation include the following: transitions to a higher level of care, critical care clinicians' cognitive load, critical care team communication, and the ICU environment's impact on diagnostic decision-making.

Higher level of care transitions. Unlike transitions of care to home or a long-term care facility, transitions to higher levels of acute care are relatively understudied, despite work showing that patients often have diagnostic discrepancies between frontline and tertiary care settings.[23,24] Emerging research shows that the characteristics of referral communication may affect the diagnosis on admission of patients to the

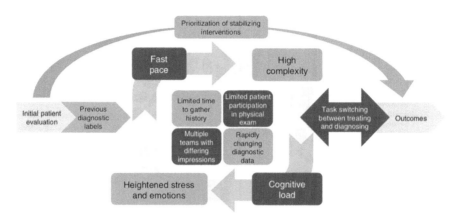

Fig. 2. Complexity and challenges in critical care diagnosis. (Adapted with permission of the American Thoracic Society. Copyright © 2021 American Thoracic Society. All rights reserved. Bergl PA, et al. Diagnostic Error in the Critically Ill: Defining the Problem and Exploring Next Steps to Advance Intensive Care Unit Safety. Ann Am Thorac Soc. 2018;15(8):903-907. Annals of the American Thoracic Society is an official journal of the American Thoracic Society. Readers are encouraged to read the entire article for the correct context at https://www.atsjournals.org/doi/full/10.1513/AnnalsATS.201801-068PS. The authors, editors, and The American Thoracic Society are not responsible for errors or omissions in adaptations.)

ICU.[25] Further work is needed to determine how information transfer, electronic health records (EHRs), professional relationships, and institutional characteristics between referring clinicians and receiving ICU teams affect diagnosis.

Critical care clinicians' cognitive load. A high cognitive load is a known risk factor for diagnostic error.[26] Clinicians practicing in the ICU perform many cognitive tasks under time pressure[3] and make hundreds of significant medical decisions per day.[27] Research using validated tools to measure information load[28] and simulation to mimic critical scenarios in the ICU[29] are needed to quantify the cognitive load of clinicians, especially during stressful situations. Simulation may also be helpful to determine the occurrence and causes of cognitive errors in diagnosis when assessing critically ill patients.[30]

Critical care team communication. Communication is at the center of much research evaluating teamwork in critical care settings.[31,32] However, little work has focused on relating the characteristics of communication with changes in the diagnostic process or diagnostic outcomes among critically ill patients. Information is conveyed in various ways (verbal vs written, in-person vs through electronic or mobile messaging) and should be investigated for its impact on diagnosis.[33,34,35] Communication during handoffs between clinicians is especially ripe for further study. Handoff practices among ICU attending physicians are heterogeneous, which are perceived by physicians to be related to inappropriate care and serious adverse events,[36] although the quality of handoffs has not been linked to diagnostic error.

The intensive care unit environment's impact on diagnostic decision-making. The critical care environment encompasses both the built physical environment of the ICU and the professional climate within which clinicians practice. In the NASEM report, the environment was emphasized as an important factor in the diagnostic process,[37] and, thus, research is needed to investigate its impact on diagnosis in critical care. In

Table 1
Research directions to understand the diagnostic process and epidemiology of diagnostic error in critical care

Potential Areas and Methods of Research	
Understanding the diagnostic process	
Transitions to higher level of care	Referral communication between referring clinicians and intensivists
	Information transfer across clinical settings
	Effect of prior diagnostic labels on ICU diagnosis
	Professional relationships' impact on the diagnostic process
	Institutional characteristics' impact on the diagnostic process
Information gathering, integration, and interpretation	Patient and family factors affecting information gathering
	Time pressure effects on information gathering and processing
	Effects of clinician cognitive load on information processing
	Contributions of subspecialty consultants to diagnosis
	Effects of clinician task-switching on diagnostic outcomes
	ICU team dynamics' contributions to diagnostic outcomes
Communication of the diagnosis	Communication of the diagnosis to the patient and family
	Communication relevant to the diagnostic process, including handoffs, clinical notes, electronic messages
Impact of the ICU environment	Contributions of the ICU built environment to the diagnostic process
	Safety climate and interpersonal relationships' impact on diagnosis
Epidemiology of diagnostic errors	
Burden of diagnostic error	Interventions to improve autopsy rates in the ICU
	Use of novel imaging technology to perform "virtual autopsies"
	Standard and validated chart review tools to determine diagnostic error
	Electronic trigger tools for identification of medical records with high likelihood of diagnostic error
Factors contributing to diagnostic error	Survey of ICU clinicians' perceptions of why diagnostic errors occur
	Qualitative interviews of patients/families and ICU clinicians
	Clinical vignette studies presenting critical care scenarios to clinicians
	Simulation studies to investigate team dynamics in diagnosis

the ICU, qualitative work shows that open, connected, and visible physical spaces encourage macrocognitive interactions among team members.[38] In a randomized simulation trial, unprofessional communication, specifically rude behavior during operating room-to-ICU handoff, resulted in the failure of the ICU team to detect and overcome diagnostic error.[39]

Diagnostic error epidemiology in critical care
Most of our knowledge of the epidemiology of diagnostic errors in critical care come from autopsy studies. Although autopsies remain a useful way to identify missed diagnoses and innovations such as the virtual autopsy[40] have increased autopsy rates beyond traditional post mortem examinations, they remain limited to patients who die. Autopsies clearly reveal the ways in which diagnostic errors can be fatal, but are less useful for studying misdiagnoses that cause harm short of death. Scientific advances in improving diagnosis will require knowledge beyond autopsies as the main source of information regarding diagnostic error in critical care (see **Table 1**).

Retrospective cohort studies performed via medical record reviews are more representative of the general ICU population[7,8,9,41]; however, the selection of study samples and the process of chart review have been variable. The relatively recent development of validated record review tools such as Singh and colleagues' Revised Safer Dx instrument,[42] which has been adapted for use in both adult and pediatric critical care settings,[7,8] should lead to more standardized reviews in future work, allowing for valid comparisons across studies. Electronic trigger tools, which mine large amounts of data to identify signals indicative of possible diagnostic error, are also a recent innovation and help to focus manual chart review efforts toward patients at high risk for error.[43]

Aside from the burden of error, factors associated with misdiagnosis also need to be identified. In addition to autopsies and chart reviews, other innovative quantitative and qualitative approaches should be used to collect richer data.[44] Even simple surveys of ICU clinicians have revealed perceived threats to accurate and timely diagnosis.[45] Qualitative observations using ethnography with audio and video review can also reveal clinician behaviors and interactions that help or hinder diagnosis.[46]

Identifying and Implementing Solutions to Improve Diagnosis

Advancing science to better diagnose critical illness
An accurate diagnosis ultimately depends on advances in biomedical science. As much as there are preventable diagnostic errors owing to failures in the diagnostic process leading to a missed or delayed diagnosis, there are also unavoidable diagnostic errors caused by inadequate scientific knowledge of illness or underdeveloped methods to diagnose disease (**Fig. 3**).[47]

The collective efforts of investigators over the decades have pushed the limits of critical care science forward, making previously unknown illness or ill-defined conditions recognizable to intensivists. Sepsis is the quintessential example of a disease—and diagnostic process—seemingly in constant flux as clinicians' understanding of the disease has evolved to keep pace with scientific discovery. Previously seen as a combination of infection and systemic inflammatory response syndrome,[48] sepsis is now widely regarded as life-threatening organ dysfunction caused by a dysregulated host response to infection.[49] New methods of detecting sepsis in the ICU have also emerged such as the use of procalcitonin levels,[50] adding to intensivists' arsenal of diagnostic tools. Further, there may be many phenotypes of sepsis, a finding that can lead to useful subcategories of diagnosis that can help to target treatment.[51]

Without losing sight of the sociotechnical components of diagnosis in critical care, we need to continue disease-specific efforts that will improve the diagnosis of unique pathophysiology in the ICU. This work includes basic and translational research into the role of biomarkers and genomics for precision diagnosis in the ICU[52,53] and clinical research on diagnostic tests and imaging to improve bedside assessment such as the use of point-of-care ultrasound examinations.[54] Similar to the evolving definitions of

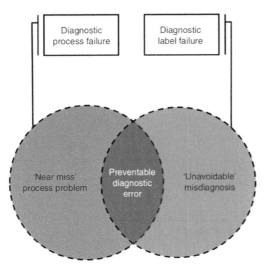

Fig. 3. Unavoidable diagnostic errors. Failures in the diagnostic process leading to failure to identify a known disease is a preventable diagnostic error. Sometimes, clinicians fail to identify a disease because of inadequate scientific knowledge, which then causes unavoidable diagnostic errors. With scientific advances over time, diagnostic errors in this category should decrease. (Reprinted with permission from De Gruyter. Newman-Toker DE. A unified conceptual model for diagnostic errors: underdiagnosis, overdiagnosis, and misdiagnosis. Diagnosis. 2014;1:43-48.)

sepsis, we need to continue to fine tune the diagnostic criteria for other critical illness such as acute respiratory distress syndrome,[55,56] develop scoring systems to accurately and reliably identify conditions relevant to ICU care such as delirium,[57] and recognize and better define emerging ICU-related conditions such as post-intensive care syndrome or "chronic critical illness".[58]

Leveraging health information technology
Diagnosis in critical care is vulnerable to human limitations. Clinicians have fallible memory, are prone to cognitive bias,[26] and communicate ineffectively.[59] Such limitations are compounded by common challenges in the ICU environment, including high workloads, constant distraction, and communication barriers.[60] Health information technology (HIT) can help clinicians to overcome or minimize these constraints[61] and should be a strong focus of research to improve diagnosis in critical care (**Table 2**).

Because HIT applications can be quite broad, it may be helpful for investigators to map potential interventions to a conceptual model of critical care diagnosis to specify which aspects of the diagnostic process are specifically being targeted.[61] Some innovations such as the EHR can have multiple applications and can assist clinicians in many aspects of diagnosis. Here, we outline specific HIT interventions applied to improve diagnosis in the ICU and potential future areas of investigation for each.

Electronic health records. The EHR has transformed clinical practice in ways both desired and unintended.[62] Future directions in research on how the EHR can further improve diagnosis in critical care thus involve not only developing new applications, but also preventing or mitigating the unintended consequences of EHR use. Pioneers in diagnostic safety have suggested many ways in which electronic clinical

Table 2
Research directions to leverage health information technology to improve diagnosis in critical care

Potential Areas of Research	
Electronic health records	
Improving clinical documentation to support diagnosis	Revise how problem lists are created and maintained
	Optimize how clinical reasoning is documented by ICU team members in clinical notes
	Develop natural language processing techniques to allow free text entry while retaining the ability to extract needed data for billing, quality improvement, and research
Improving data organization and presentation to clinicians	Optimize clinical summarization functions of the EHR
	Develop graphical data visualizations optimized to ease clinicians' cognitive load
Interoperability and data standards	Increase interoperability of EHR systems within and across organizations for better information flow
Feedback functions	Develop electronic tools to deliver automated clinician feedback on patients' changing diagnoses
Telemedicine	
Configuration of telemedicine care model	Determine optimal characteristics of critical care providers, recipient ICUs, patient populations to maximize benefits to diagnosis
	Develop implementation structures and workflows to best support diagnosis
Integration of other HIT interventions into telemedicine	Investigate how AI and machine learning can be used to improve diagnosis, leveraging the large volumes of data generated by telemedicine
Clinical Decision Support Systems	
Traditional CDSS[a]	Redesign traditional CDSSs to improve utility in assisting with diagnosis, improve usability, and prevent alert fatigue among clinicians
Integration of other HIT interventions with CDSS	Study the effects of embedding clinical care pathways into CDSSs on the diagnostic process
	Investigate the impact of AI and machine learning-powered CDSSs on diagnostic outcomes
CDSS and ICU workflow	Optimize the manner in which CDSS are incorporated into ICU workflows

(continued on next page)

Table 2 (*continued*)	
Potential Areas of Research	
Artificial Intelligence and machine learning	
Development and training of AI systems	Identify specific diagnostic scenarios most appropriate for interventions using AI and machine learning Determine appropriate ICU datasets for training AI systems tailored to specific diagnostic goals Identify and correct for health care disparities that may be included in training datasets
Validation of diagnostic output	Validate AI systems' diagnostic output under realistic or real-world ICU conditions
AI and ICU workflow	Study how AI systems can be deployed most effectively within ICU workflows Optimize the balance between decision support and clinician autonomy in diagnostic decision-making

Abbreviations: AI, artificial intelligence; CDSS, clinical decision support systems; EHR, electronic health record; HIT, health information technology.

[a] Traditional CDSS includes simple alerts, reminders, order sets, medical calculators, and care summary dashboards.

documentation can be improved to support diagnosis,[34,62] which in turn need to be studied for applicability to the critical care setting. These include revising how problem lists are created and updated, as well as ensuring that clinical reasoning is documented in the medical record. Natural language processing should allow extraction of structured data elements from free text documentation for billing, quality improvement, and clinical research.[63] Research is also needed to determine optimal ways of summarizing and presenting information to clinicians to ease cognitive load and minimize bias in data interpretation.[64] Because critical care patients are almost always referred to the ICU from a different clinical setting, efforts to increase interoperability of EHRs between organizations should be a priority to ensure the smooth transfer of critical information between institutions.[65] The EHR's ability to provide feedback on diagnostic performance is also understudied—there is an opportunity to develop automated feedback systems so that clinicians can be informed of patients' changing diagnoses even after transfer out of the ICU.[66]

Telemedicine in critical care. Telemedicine—the use of medical information exchanged using electronic communication—is rapidly becoming an established care delivery model in critical care because it extends ICU expertise.[67] Telemedicine is associated with lower ICU and hospital mortality rates.[68,69] However, little work has been performed to determine the impact of telemedicine on diagnosis. There is literature showing that the implementation of a tele-ICU is associated with improved teamwork and safety climate,[70] which can potentially translate into better diagnosis; however, optimal characteristics of critical care providers, recipient ICUs, patient populations, and implementation structures and workflows have not been identified.[68,69] Telemedicine will likely be a fixture of ICU care in the future; therefore, dedicated research is needed to delineate how this care model affects the diagnostic process.

Implementing other types of HIT applications such as clinical decision support and artificial intelligence (AI) onto a telemedicine platform is also a promising new area of investigation.[71]

Clinical decision support. A clinical decision support system (CDSS) is any electronic system designed to aid directly in clinical decision-making, wherein the characteristics of individual patients are used to generate patient-specific recommendations presented to clinicians for consideration.[72] CDSSs can assist critical care clinicians in a wide range of diagnostic activities, from the simple selection of diagnostic tests to support for resolving diagnostic dilemmas.[73] Most CDSSs are now embedded within and deployed using the EHR. Traditional examples include alerts, reminders, order sets, medical calculators, and care summary dashboards. Over time, CDSSs have included information retrieval tools (infobuttons) available alongside clinical information to aid clinicians in the search and retrieval of patient- and context-specific knowledge.[74] CDSSs have also incorporated clinical care pathways, which are structured multidisciplinary plans of care operationalizing evidence-based guidelines for the criteria-based implementation of standard diagnosis and management.[75] Although several systematic reviews have shown evidence of improved implementation of health care processes (specifically, ordering appropriate diagnostic tests) in diverse clinical settings using CDSS,[72,75,76] there remains minimal evidence of its impact on diagnostic outcomes, especially among critically ill patients. In addition to improving diagnostic algorithms and the medical knowledge databases that underpin CDSSs, future directions should also include investigations into improving clinician acceptance and devising optimal ways to integrate these systems into ICU clinical workflows.[77]

Artificial intelligence and machine learning. The advanced analytical methods of AI systems and machine learning techniques (a subset of AI)—where computers process large amounts of data to learn from examples, rather than being preprogrammed with rules based on human inputs—have the potential to fundamentally change medical practice.[78] In the data-intensive environment of the ICU, such systems can assist clinicians in efficiently processing large volumes of information to make an expeditious and accurate diagnosis. The most practical impact of AI on critical care diagnosis will likely be through machine learning-powered CDSSs designed to be used interactively by clinicians at the bedside. Early studies have shown promising results related to the prediction of physiologic instability and early detection of conditions such as sepsis, acute respiratory distress syndrome, pulmonary embolism, and acute kidney injury.[79,80] However, a recent systematic review showed sparse evidence of association between machine learning-based CDSSs and diagnostic performance owing to a small sample size, unclear risk of study bias, lack of consideration of human factors, and lack of studies evaluating these systems under real-world conditions.[81] Thus, although these innovative techniques hold immense promise, future research will need to address specific barriers to progress in this field. For instance, machine learning models depend on gold standards in training data with which to compare subsequent previously unseen data. This aspect of machine learning presents a problem in critical care because much of ICU practice is highly subjective, multiple diagnostic pathways are often reasonable, and few clinical decisions are unequivocally right.[79] AI systems also have difficulty drawing inferences from limited data, making them less useful for identifying rare or unusual conditions.[82] Furthermore, datasets may contain data reflecting health care disparities in the provision of systematically worse care for vulnerable groups, which AI systems can then erroneously learn.[83] Researchers must thus judiciously choose particular aspects of critical care diagnosis that are most suited to AI support and select appropriate training datasets while taking precautions to protect against unintended bias. Aside from overcoming these inherent issues in AI system training and function, investigators must also study how best to incorporate these tools into the ICU, ensuring that clinicians trust in the performance of the system without encouraging decision-making passivity and preventing alert fatigue.[84]

Finally, the thoughtful implementation of HIT into complex clinical workflows and environments is just as important as the programmed functions of the HIT application itself. Poorly implemented initiatives using HIT can be more harmful than not using HIT at all.[85] For successful implementation and maximum benefit, investigators should strive to embed human factors engineering in the user-centered design of HIT interventions[86] to create useable and sustainable systems. A useful framework to consider is Singh and Sittig's Health IT Safety Framework,[87] which provides a guide to considering the many sociotechnical dimensions of implementing HIT into complex health care systems.

Improving Team Cognition and Teamwork

One of the top recommendations of the NASEM report was to improve teamwork in the diagnostic process.[88] This recommendation is a welcome departure from the classic thinking that physicians are solely responsible for diagnosis. The literature is replete with the known benefits of teamwork in medicine[89] and specifically in the ICU,[90] where teamwork has improved both clinical processes and patient outcomes. Despite this awareness, there are few studies investigating how to optimize teamwork to improve critical care diagnosis. We are only beginning to understand the role of nurses,[91] allied medical professionals,[92] and subspecialty consultants in diagnosis,[93] but further research is needed to determine how to maximize their contributions given each member's specific role in critical care. Early studies have also revealed the importance of developing shared mental models across ICU team members to deliver appropriate care.[94,95] Researchers need to build on this work to better understand how different ways of communicating affect mental model creation across an interprofessional group[33,35,36] and leverage known principles and methods in human factors and cognitive psychology to support interventions that will help teams to quickly achieve a shared patient understanding. In the ICU, certain team tasks are high yield for improving diagnosis. For example, daily team rounds seem to be an obvious locus of day-to-day ICU team collaboration and decision-making,[96] whereas critical patient events wherein multiple team members are helping to troubleshoot at the bedside present situations where urgent team decisions and actions need to be made.[97] Researchers may do well to focus on these low-hanging fruit of ICU scenarios ripe for study to improve team diagnosis. Finally, in addition to determining the effects of teamwork interventions on patient outcomes such as mortality, investigators need to shift their attention to diagnosis-relevant outcomes of teamwork, such as accuracy and timeliness of diagnosis and the occurrence of diagnosis-related harm.

Including Patients and Families in the Diagnostic Process

Patient-centered care is defined as care that is respectful of and responsive to individual patients' and families' preferences, needs, and values.[98] Major professional critical care organizations have endorsed this approach for the past decade or more, suggesting that patient and family involvement can profoundly influence clinical decisions and patient outcomes in the ICU.[99] Although most ICUs have incorporated patient-centered and family-centered care,[99,100] we have yet to explore how shared decision making in diagnosis can be effectively integrated into this model. The concept of patient-centered diagnosis is relatively new, and it is distinguished from shared decision-making for treatment by (1) the greater uncertainty in the diagnostic process, (2) the patient's and clinician's tolerance for uncertainty, (3) benefits and harms of diagnostic tests that are more difficult to quantify, and (4) the more iterative nature of diagnostic decision-making.[101] Research in this area should focus on how to incorporate shared diagnostic decision-making with families during common activities in the ICU such as family-centered rounds and family conferences. Work is needed to determine optimal ways for clinicians to convey information on the benefits and risks of testing in light of critical illness and eliciting patients' and families' preferences and risk tolerance.[101]

SUMMARY

Research to improve diagnosis in critical care medicine has accelerated with an increasing awareness of the burden and harms of diagnostic error among critically ill patients. However, much work remains to fully elucidate the diagnostic process in critical care, which is fundamental to understanding how diagnostic errors occur in the ICU. Interdisciplinary research is needed to investigate the many potential interventions to improve diagnostic outcomes and prevent diagnostic-error related harm in this population. To make significant progress toward diagnostic excellence, we need to adopt a balanced strategy of continued biomedical discovery while addressing the complex care delivery systems underpinning the diagnosis of critical illness.

CLINICS CARE POINTS

- Research to improve diagnosis in critical care medicine has accelerated with increasing awareness of the burden and harms of diagnostic error among critically ill patients.
- Much work remains to fully elucidate the diagnostic process in critical care, which is fundamental to understanding how diagnostic errors occur in the ICU.
- To achieve diagnostic excellence, interdisciplinary research is needed, adopting a balanced strategy of continued biomedical discovery while addressing the complex care delivery systems underpinning the diagnosis of critical illness.

REFERENCES

1. Bergl PA, Nanchal RS, Singh H. Diagnostic error in the critically ill: defining the problem and exploring next steps to advance intensive care unit safety. Ann Am Thorac Soc 2018;15(8):903–7.
2. Newman-Toker DE, Pham J, Winters BD, et al. Diagnostic errors in critical care settings – managing information overload. ICU Manag Summer 2009;9(2):6–11.
3. Shaw M, Singh S. Complex clinical reasoning in the critical care unit - difficulties, pitfalls and adaptive strategies. Int J Clin Pract 2015;69(4):396–400.
4. Moss M, Good VS, Gozal D, et al. An official critical care societies collaborative statement: burnout syndrome in critical care healthcare professionals: a call for action. Crit Care Med 2016;44(7):1414–21.
5. Winters B, Custer J, Galvagno SM, et al. Diagnostic errors in the intensive care unit: a systematic review of autopsy studies. BMJ Qual Saf 2012;21(11):894–902.
6. Custer JW, Winters BD, Goode V, et al. Diagnostic errors in the pediatric and neonatal ICU: a systematic review. Pediatr Crit Care Med 2015;16(1):29–36.

7. Bergl PA, Taneja A, El-Kareh R, et al. Frequency, risk factors, causes, and consequences of diagnostic errors in critically ill medical patients: a retrospective cohort study. Crit Care Med 2019;47(11):e902–10.

8. Cifra CL, Ten Eyck P, Dawson JD, et al. Factors associated with diagnostic error on admission to a PICU: a pilot study. Pediatr Crit Care Med 2020;21(5):e311–5.

9. Shafer GJ, Suresh G. Diagnostic errors in the neonatal intensive care unit: a case series. AJP Rep 2018;8(4):e379–83.

10. National Academies of Sciences, Engineering, and Medicine. A research agenda for the diagnostic process and diagnostic error. In: Balogh EP, Miller BT, Ball JR, editors. Improving diagnosis in health care. Washington, DC: The National Academies Press; 2015. p. 343–54.

11. Zwaan L, Singh H. Diagnostic error in hospitals: finding forests not just the big trees. BMJ Qual Saf 2020;29(12):961–4.

12. Zwaan L, El-Kareh R, Meyer AND, et al. Advancing diagnostic safety research: results of a systematic research priority setting exercise. J Gen Intern Med 2021. Published online February 9, 2021. doi: 10.1007/s11606-020-06428-3.

13. Coalition to Improve Diagnosis. Society to improve diagnosis in medicine. Available at: https://www.improvediagnosis.org/coalition/. Accessed January 12, 2021.

14. Lujan BR. Improving diagnosis in medicine act of 2019. Published November 12, 2019. Available at: https://www.congress.gov/bill/116th-congress/house-bill/5014/text. Accessed January 12, 2021.

15. Cifra CL, Custer JW, Singh H, et al. Diagnostic errors in pediatric critical care: a systematic review. Pediatr Crit Care Med 2021. Published online April 8, 2021. doi: 10.1097/PCC.0000000000002735.

16. Cifra CL, Jones KL, Ascenzi JA, et al. Diagnostic errors in a PICU: insights from the morbidity and mortality conference. Pediatr Crit Care Med 2015;16(5): 468–76.

17. Saber Tehrani AS, Lee H, Mathews SC, et al. 25-Year summary of US malpractice claims for diagnostic errors 1986-2010: an analysis from the National Practitioner Data Bank. BMJ Qual Saf 2013;22(8):672–80.

18. Gupta A, Snyder A, Kachalia A, et al. Malpractice claims related to diagnostic errors in the hospital. BMJ Qual Saf 2017;27(1). bmjqs-2017-006774.

19. Giardina TD, Haskell H, Menon S, et al. Learning from patients' experiences related to diagnostic errors is essential for progress in patient safety. Health Aff Proj Hope 2018;37(11):1821–7.

20. Kaur AP, Levinson AT, Monteiro JFG, et al. The impact of errors on healthcare professionals in the critical care setting. J Crit Care 2019;52:16–21.

21. Wu AW, Steckelberg RC. Medical error, incident investigation and the second victim: doing better but feeling worse? BMJ Qual Saf 2012;21(4):267–70.

22. National Academies of Sciences, Engineering, and Medicine. The diagnostic process. In: Balogh EP, Miller BT, Ball JR, editors. Improving diagnosis in health care. Washington, DC: The National Academies Press; 2015. p. 31–80.

23. Philpot C, Day S, Marcdante K, et al. Pediatric interhospital transport: diagnostic discordance and hospital mortality. Pediatr Crit Care Med 2008;9(1):15–9.

24. Usher M, Sahni N, Herrigel D, et al. Diagnostic discordance, health information exchange, and inter-hospital transfer outcomes: a population study. J Gen Intern Med 2018;33(9):1447–53.

25. Cifra CL, Dukes KC, Ayres BS, et al. Referral communication for pediatric intensive care unit admission and the diagnosis of critically ill children: a pilot ethnography. J Crit Care 2021;63:246–9.

26. Croskerry P. The importance of cognitive errors in diagnosis and strategies to minimize them. Acad Med J Assoc Am Med Coll 2003;78(8):775–80.
27. McKenzie MS, Auriemma CL, Olenik J, et al. An observational study of decision making by medical intensivists. Crit Care Med 2015;43(8):1660–8.
28. Friedman ML, McBride ME. Changes in cognitive function after pediatric intensive care unit rounds: a prospective study. Diagnosis 2016;3(3):123–8.
29. Pawar S, Jacques T, Deshpande K, et al. Evaluation of cognitive load and emotional states during multidisciplinary critical care simulation sessions. BMJ Simul Technol Enhanc Learn 2018;4(2):87–91.
30. Prakash S, Bihari S, Need P, et al. Immersive high fidelity simulation of critically ill patients to study cognitive errors: a pilot study. BMC Med Educ 2017;17(1):36.
31. Stocker M, Pilgrim SB, Burmester M, et al. Interprofessional team management in pediatric critical care: some challenges and possible solutions. J Multidiscip Healthc 2016;9:47–58.
32. Dietz AS, Pronovost PJ, Mendez-Tellez PA, et al. A systematic review of teamwork in the intensive care unit: what do we know about teamwork, team tasks, and improvement strategies? J Crit Care 2014;29(6):908–14.
33. Collins SA, Bakken S, Vawdrey DK, et al. Clinician preferences for verbal communication compared to EHR documentation in the ICU. Appl Clin Inform 2011;2(2):190–201.
34. Schiff GD, Bates DW. Can electronic clinical documentation help prevent diagnostic errors? N Engl J Med 2010;362(12):1066–9.
35. Martin G, Khajuria A, Arora S, et al. The impact of mobile technology on teamwork and communication in hospitals: a systematic review. JAMIA 2019;26(4):339–55.
36. Lane-Fall MB, Collard ML, Turnbull AE, et al. ICU attending handoff practices: results from a National Survey of Academic Intensivists. Crit Care Med 2016;44(4):690–8.
37. National Academies of Sciences, Engineering, and Medicine. Organizational characteristics, the physical environment, and the diagnostic process: improving learning, culture, and the work system. In: Balogh EP, Miller BT, Ball JR, editors. Improving diagnosis in health care. Washington, DC: The National Academies Press; 2015. p. 263–305.
38. O'Hara S, Klar RT, Patterson ES, et al. Macrocognition in the healthcare built environment (mHCBE): a focused ethnographic study of "neighborhoods" in a pediatric intensive care unit. HERD 2018;11(2):104–23.
39. Avesar M, Erez A, Essakow J, et al. The effect of rudeness on challenging diagnostic error: a randomized controlled simulation trial. Crit Care Med 2019;47(1).
40. Wichmann D, Obbelode F, Vogel H, et al. Virtual autopsy as an alternative to traditional medical autopsy in the intensive care unit: a prospective cohort study. Ann Intern Med 2012;156(2):123–30.
41. Davalos MC, Samuels K, Meyer AND, et al. Finding diagnostic errors in children admitted to the PICU. Pediatr Crit Care Med 2017;18(3):265–71.
42. Singh H, Khanna A, Spitzmueller C, et al. Recommendations for using the Revised Safer Dx Instrument to help measure and improve diagnostic safety. Diagnosis 2019;6(4):315–23.
43. Murphy DR, Meyer AN, Sittig DF, et al. Application of electronic trigger tools to identify targets for improving diagnostic safety. BMJ Qual Saf 2019;28(2):151–9.
44. Zwaan L, Singh H. The challenges in defining and measuring diagnostic error. Diagnosis 2015;2(2):97–103.

45. Bhat PN, Costello JM, Aiyagari R, et al. Diagnostic errors in paediatric cardiac intensive care. Cardiol Young 2018;28(5):675–82.
46. Su L, Kaplan S, Waller M. Video review produces insight into diagnostic errors. Diagnosis 2015;2(1):eA29–30.
47. Newman-Toker DE. A unified conceptual model for diagnostic errors: underdiagnosis, overdiagnosis, and misdiagnosis. Diagnosis 2014;1:43–8.
48. American College of Chest Physicians/Society of Critical Care Medicine Consensus Conference: definitions for sepsis and organ failure and guidelines for the use of innovative therapies in sepsis. Crit Care Med 1992;20(6):864–74.
49. Singer M, Deutschman CS, Seymour CW, et al. The third international consensus definitions for sepsis and septic shock (Sepsis-3). JAMA 2016;315(8):801–10.
50. Patnaik R, Azim A, Mishra P. Should serial monitoring of procalcitonin be done routinely in critically ill patients of ICU: a systematic review and meta-analysis. J Anaesthesiol Clin Pharmacol 2020;36(4):458–64.
51. Seymour CW, Kennedy JN, Wang S, et al. Derivation, validation, and potential treatment implications of novel clinical phenotypes for sepsis. JAMA 2019;321(20):2003–17.
52. Sarma A, Calfee CS, Ware LB. Biomarkers and precision medicine: state of the art. Crit Care Clin 2020;36(1):155–65.
53. French CE, Delon I, Dolling H, et al. Whole genome sequencing reveals that genetic conditions are frequent in intensively ill children. Intensive Care Med 2019;45(5):627–36.
54. Campbell SJ, Bechara R, Islam S. Point-of-care ultrasound in the intensive care unit. Clin Chest Med 2018;39(1):79–97.
55. Fan E, Brodie D, Slutsky AS. Acute respiratory distress syndrome: advances in diagnosis and treatment. JAMA 2018;319(7):698–710.
56. Khemani RG, Smith LS, Zimmerman JJ, et al, Pediatric Acute Lung Injury Consensus Conference Group. Pediatric acute respiratory distress syndrome: definition, incidence, and epidemiology: proceedings from the Pediatric Acute Lung Injury Consensus Conference. Pediatr Crit Care Med 2015;16(5 Suppl 1):S23–40.
57. Smith HAB, Boyd J, Fuchs DC, et al. Diagnosing delirium in critically ill children: validity and reliability of the pediatric confusion assessment method for the intensive care unit. Crit Care Med 2011;39(1):150–7.
58. Inoue S, Hatakeyama J, Kondo Y, et al. Post-intensive care syndrome: its pathophysiology, prevention, and future directions. Acute Med Surg 2019;6(3):233–46.
59. Grant M. Resolving communication challenges in the intensive care unit. AACN Adv Crit Care 2015;26(2):123–30.
60. Montgomery VL. Effect of fatigue, workload, and environment on patient safety in the pediatric intensive care unit. Pediatr Crit Care Med 2007;8(2 Suppl):S11–6.
61. El-Kareh R, Hasan O, Schiff GD. Use of health information technology to reduce diagnostic errors. BMJ Qual Saf 2013;22(Suppl 2):ii40–51.
62. Graber ML, Byrne C, Johnston D. The impact of electronic health records on diagnosis. Diagnosis 2017;4(4):211–23.
63. Meystre S, Haug P. Improving the sensitivity of the problem list in an intensive care unit by using natural language processing. AMIA Symp 2006;2006:554–8.

64. Wright MC, Dunbar S, Macpherson BC, et al. Toward designing information display to support critical care. A qualitative contextual evaluation and visioning effort. Appl Clin Inform 2016;7(4):912–29.
65. Janett RS, Yeracaris PP. Electronic medical records in the American health system: challenges and lessons learned. Cienc Saude Coletiva 2020;25(4): 1293–304.
66. Shenvi EC, Feupe SF, Yang H, et al. "Closing the loop": a mixed-methods study about resident learning from outcome feedback after patient handoffs. Diagnosis 2018;5(4):235–42.
67. Herasevich V, Subramanian S. Tele-ICU technologies. Crit Care Clin 2019;35(3): 427–38.
68. Wilcox ME, Adhikari NKJ. The effect of telemedicine in critically ill patients: systematic review and meta-analysis. Crit Care Lond Engl 2012;16(4):R127.
69. Chen J, Sun D, Yang W, et al. Clinical and economic outcomes of telemedicine programs in the intensive care unit: a systematic review and meta-analysis. J Intensive Care Med 2018;33(7):383–93.
70. Chu-Weininger MYL, Wueste L, Lucke JF, et al. The impact of a tele-ICU on provider attitudes about teamwork and safety climate. Qual Saf Health Care 2010; 19(6):e39.
71. Kindle RD, Badawi O, Celi LA, et al. Intensive care unit telemedicine in the era of big data, artificial intelligence, and computer clinical decision support systems. Crit Care Clin 2019;35(3):483–95.
72. Bright TJ, Wong A, Dhurjati R, et al. Effect of clinical decision-support systems: a systematic review. Ann Intern Med 2012;157(1):29–43.
73. Mack EH, Wheeler DS, Embi PJ. Clinical decision support systems in the pediatric intensive care unit. Pediatr Crit Care Med 2009;10(1):23–8.
74. Cook DA, Teixeira MT, Heale BS, et al. Context-sensitive decision support (infobuttons) in electronic health records: a systematic review. JAMIA 2017;24(2): 460–8.
75. Neame MT, Chacko J, Surace AE, et al. A systematic review of the effects of implementing clinical pathways supported by health information technologies. JAMIA 2019;26(4):356–63.
76. Main C, Moxham T, Wyatt JC, et al. Computerised decision support systems in order communication for diagnostic, screening or monitoring test ordering: systematic reviews of the effects and cost-effectiveness of systems. Health Technol Assess Winch Engl 2010;14(48):1–227.
77. Miller RA. Computer-assisted diagnostic decision support: history, challenges, and possible paths forward. Adv Health Sci Educ Theor Pract 2009;14(Suppl 1):89–106.
78. Clinical decision support systems. Available at: https://psnet.ahrq.gov/primer/clinical-decision-support-systems. Accessed April 19, 2021.
79. Gutierrez G. Artificial intelligence in the intensive care unit. Crit Care Lond Engl 2020;24(1):101.
80. Despins LA. Automated deterioration detection using electronic medical record data in intensive care unit patients: a systematic review. Comput Inform Nurs CIN 2018;36(7):323–30.
81. Vasey B, Ursprung S, Beddoe B, et al. Association of clinician diagnostic performance with machine learning-based decision support systems: a systematic review. JAMA Netw Open 2021;4(3):e211276.
82. Desai AN. Artificial intelligence: promise, pitfalls, and perspective. JAMA 2020; 323(24):2448–9.

83. Rajkomar A, Dean J, Kohane I. Machine learning in medicine. N Engl J Med 2019;380(14):1347–58.
84. Yu K-H, Kohane IS. Framing the challenges of artificial intelligence in medicine. BMJ Qual Saf 2019;28(3):238–41.
85. Coiera E, Ash J, Berg M. The unintended consequences of health information technology revisited. Yearb Med Inform 2016;1:163–9.
86. Carayon P, Hoonakker P. Human factors and usability for health information technology: old and new challenges. Yearb Med Inform 2019;28(1):71–7.
87. Singh H, Sittig DF. Measuring and improving patient safety through health information technology: the Health IT Safety Framework. BMJ Qual Saf 2016;25(4):226–32.
88. National Academies of Sciences, Engineering, and Medicine. Diagnostic team members and tasks: improving patient engagement and healthcare professional education and training in diagnosis. In: Balogh EP, Miller BT, Ball JR, editors. Improving diagnosis in health care. Washington, DC: The National Academies Press; 2015. p. 145–216.
89. Schmutz JB, Meier LL, Manser T. How effective is teamwork really? The relationship between teamwork and performance in healthcare teams: a systematic review and meta-analysis. BMJ Open 2019;9(9):e028280.
90. Wheelan SA, Burchill CN, Tilin F. The link between teamwork and patients' outcomes in intensive care units. Am J Crit Care 2003;12(6):527–34.
91. Gleason KT, Davidson PM, Tanner EK, et al. Defining the critical role of nurses in diagnostic error prevention: a conceptual framework and a call to action. Diagnosis 2017;4(4):201–10.
92. Thomas DB, Newman-Toker DE. Diagnosis is a team sport - partnering with allied health professionals to reduce diagnostic errors: a case study on the role of a vestibular therapist in diagnosing dizziness. Diagnosis 2016;3(2):49–59.
93. Braiteh F, El Osta B, Palmer JL, et al. Characteristics, findings, and outcomes of palliative care inpatient consultations at a comprehensive cancer center. J Palliat Med 2007;10(4):948–55.
94. Custer JW, White E, Fackler JC, et al. A qualitative study of expert and team cognition on complex patients in the pediatric intensive care unit. Pediatr Crit Care Med 2012;13(3):278–84.
95. Fackler JC, Watts C, Grome A, et al. Critical care physician cognitive task analysis: an exploratory study. Crit Care Lond Engl 2009;13(2):R33.
96. Ervin JN, Kahn JM, Cohen TR, et al. Teamwork in the intensive care unit. Am Psychol 2018;73(4):468–77.
97. Tschan F, Semmer N, Gurtner A, et al. Explicit reasoning, confirmation bias, and illusory transactive memory: a simulation study of group medical decision making. Small Group Res 2009;40:271–300.
98. Catalyst N. What is patient-centered care? NEJM Catal January 1, 2017. Available at: https://catalyst.nejm.org/doi/full/10.1056/CAT.17.0559. Accessed April 20, 2021.
99. Meert KL, Clark J, Eggly S. Family-centered care in the pediatric intensive care unit. Pediatr Clin North Am 2013;60(3):761–72.
100. Ludmir J, Netzer G. Family-centered care in the intensive care unit-what does best practice tell us? Semin Respir Crit Care Med 2019;40(5):648–54.
101. Berger ZD, Brito JP, Ospina NS, et al. Patient centred diagnosis: sharing diagnostic decisions with patients in clinical practice. BMJ 2017;359:j4218.

Moving?

Make sure your subscription moves with you!

To notify us of your new address, find your **Clinics Account Number** (located on your mailing label above your name), and contact customer service at:

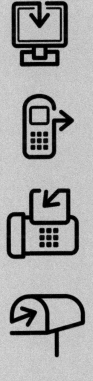

Email: **journalscustomerservice-usa@elsevier.com**

800-654-2452 (subscribers in the U.S. & Canada)
314-447-8871 (subscribers outside of the U.S. & Canada)

Fax number: 314-447-8029

Elsevier Health Sciences Division
Subscription Customer Service
3251 Riverport Lane
Maryland Heights, MO 63043

ELSEVIER